Exercise Is Fun!

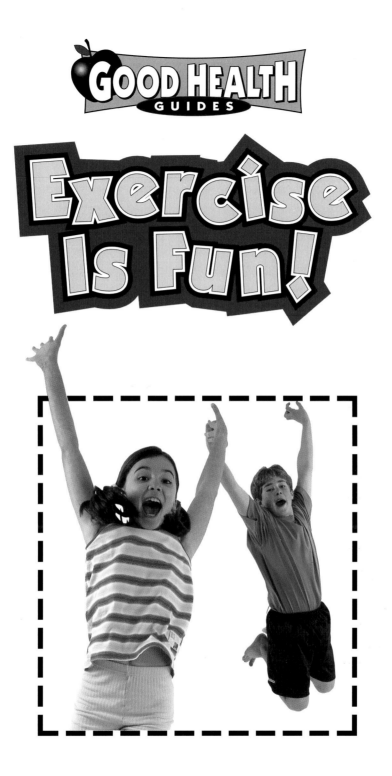

PUBLISHER'S NOTE:
It is advisable for young children to exercise with adult supervision. In addition, if there is any doubt about the state of a child's health, particularly where there is a physical disability or an asthmatic condition, please consult with a doctor as to whether the exercises presented in this book are suitable. On no account should an exercise sequence be continued if pain or strain is experienced.

For a free color catalog describing Gareth Stevens' list of high-quality books and multimedia programs, call 1-800-542-2595 (USA) or 1-800-461-9120 (Canada). Gareth Stevens Publishing's Fax: (414) 225-0377. See our catalog, too, on the World Wide Web: gsinc.com

Library of Congress Cataloging-in-Publication Data

Green, Tamara, 1945-
Exercise is fun! / by Tamara Green.
p. cm. — (Good health guides)
Includes bibliographical references and index.
Summary: Explains the benefits of physical activity and presents a series of exercises that can be done by individuals or in a group.
ISBN 0-8368-2180-7 (lib. bdg.)
1. Exercise for children—Juvenile literature. 2. Exercise—Juvenile literature. 3. Physical fitness—Juvenile literature. [1. Exercise. 2. Physical fitness.] I. Title. II. Series: Good health guides (Milwaukee, WI)
RJ133.G74 1998
613.7'1—dc21 98-24236

This North American edition first published in 1998 by
Gareth Stevens Publishing
1555 North RiverCenter Drive, Suite 201
Milwaukee, Wisconsin 53212 USA

Consultants: Dr. Martin Wright, general practitioner, and Sharon Cooper, physical education instructor
Photography: Kostas Grivas
Additional photography and artwork: Sue Baker/Deidre Bleeze
U.K. series editor: Tamara Green
Design: Marilyn Franks

U.S. series editor: Dorothy L. Gibbs
Editorial assistants: Mary Dykstra and Diane Laska

Printed in Mexico

1 2 3 4 5 6 7 8 9 02 01 00 99 98

Good Health Guides

Exercise Is Fun!

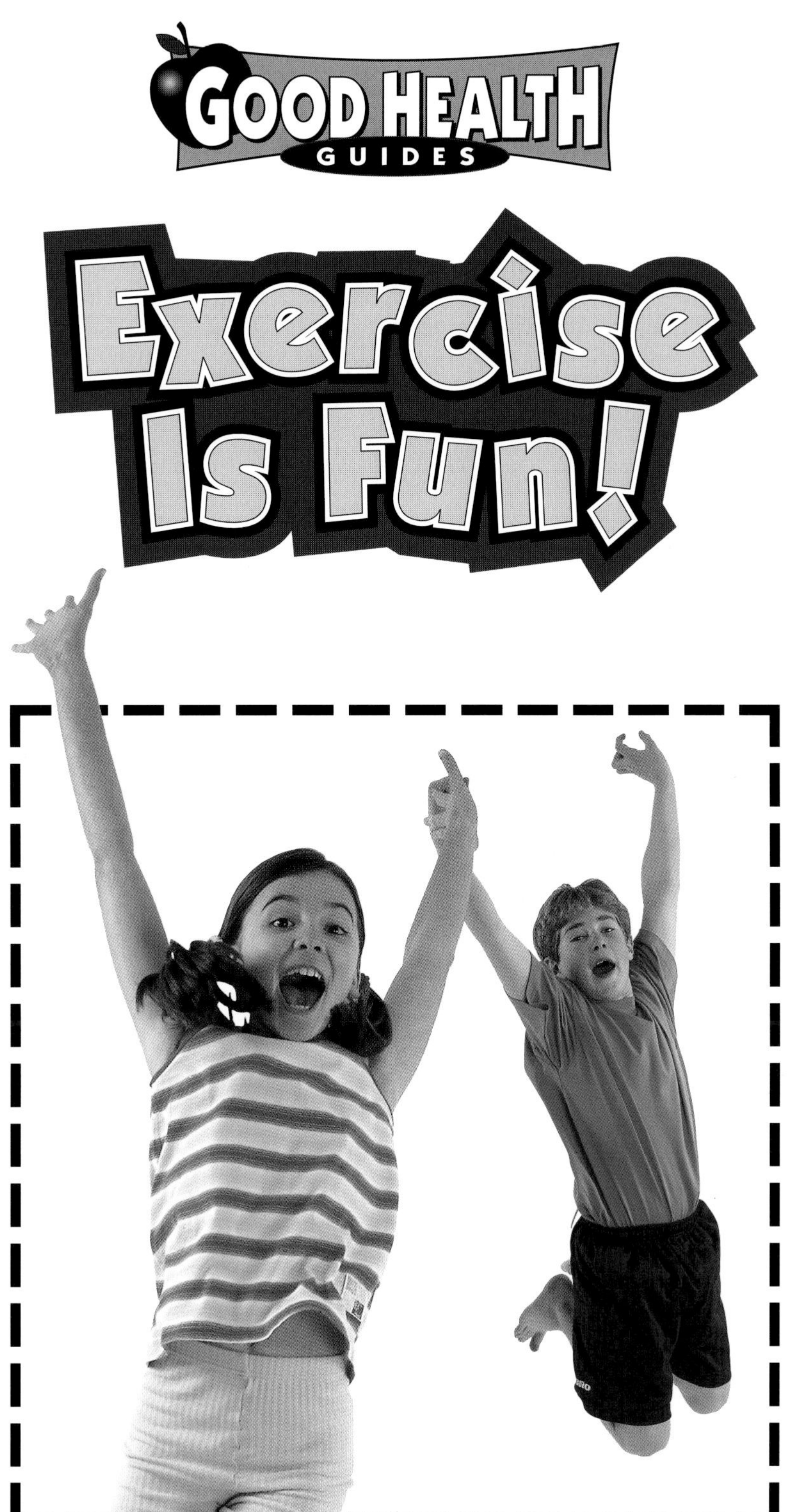

Tamara Green

Gareth Stevens Publishing
MILWAUKEE

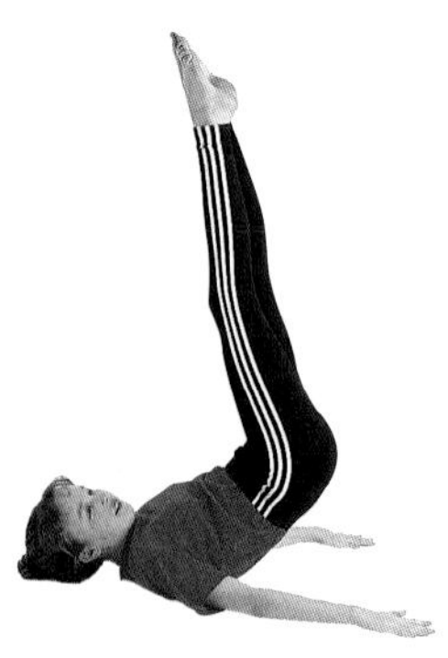

Contents

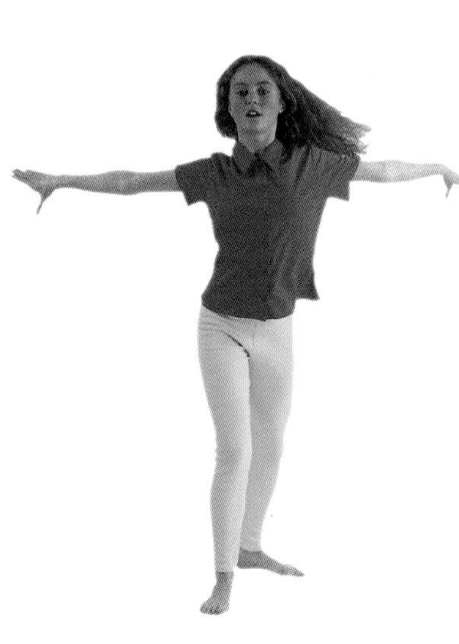

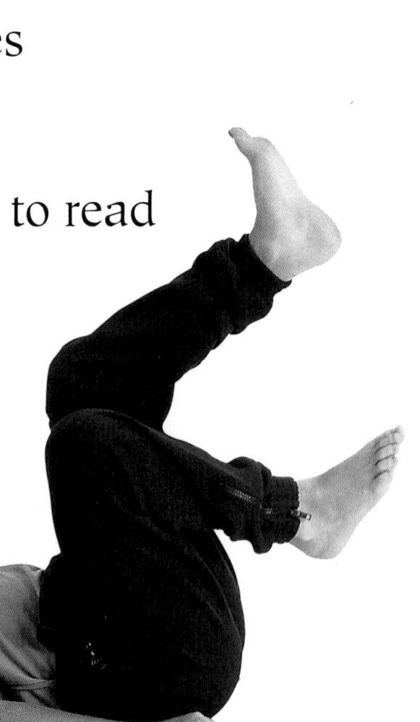

Introduction

Do you like sports and exercise? Or would you admit to being a couch potato, preferring to sit slouched in front of the TV or staring at a computer screen for hours on end?

Either way, this book is for you. It is designed for boys and girls who already enjoy keeping physically fit as well as for those who need a little encouragement to start exercising.

Why is exercise so important? Looking good and feeling good don't often come naturally. You have to work at them, and exercise is one of the ways to do it.

If you try the exercises on the following pages, you will discover that certain routines, practiced over time, make you look and feel better. Some can strengthen lung function; others tone muscles or improve posture. Exercise can help keep your mind alert, too. Each routine in this book also offers a challenge for boys and girls who are already very fit.

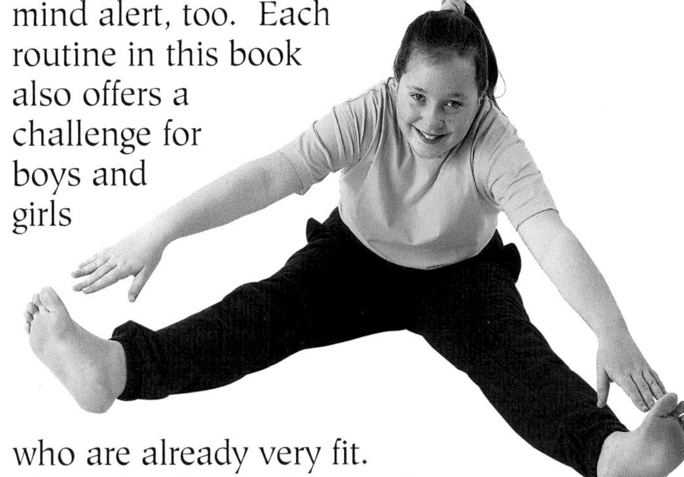

Exercise doesn't have to be boring. Some of the workouts presented in this book, such as animal antics and making faces, are lots of fun. You don't need expensive equipment either, and any kind of loose-fitting clothing will do. Best of all, you can exercise in bare feet if you're on a level, nonslip floor. Just be sure not to exercise right after a meal, and slow down, or stop exercising, if you feel yourself straining. Always take a few minutes after exercising to relax and cool down.

Whatever shape you're in, why not spend just five minutes each day discovering that EXERCISE IS FUN! You might get a little hot and sweaty, but working out is very cool!

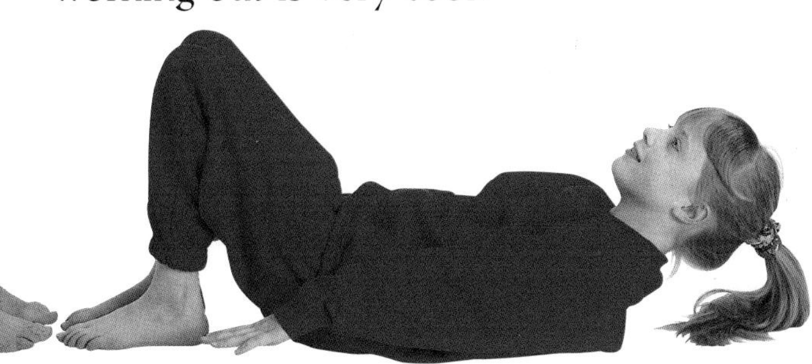

Breathing in, breathing out

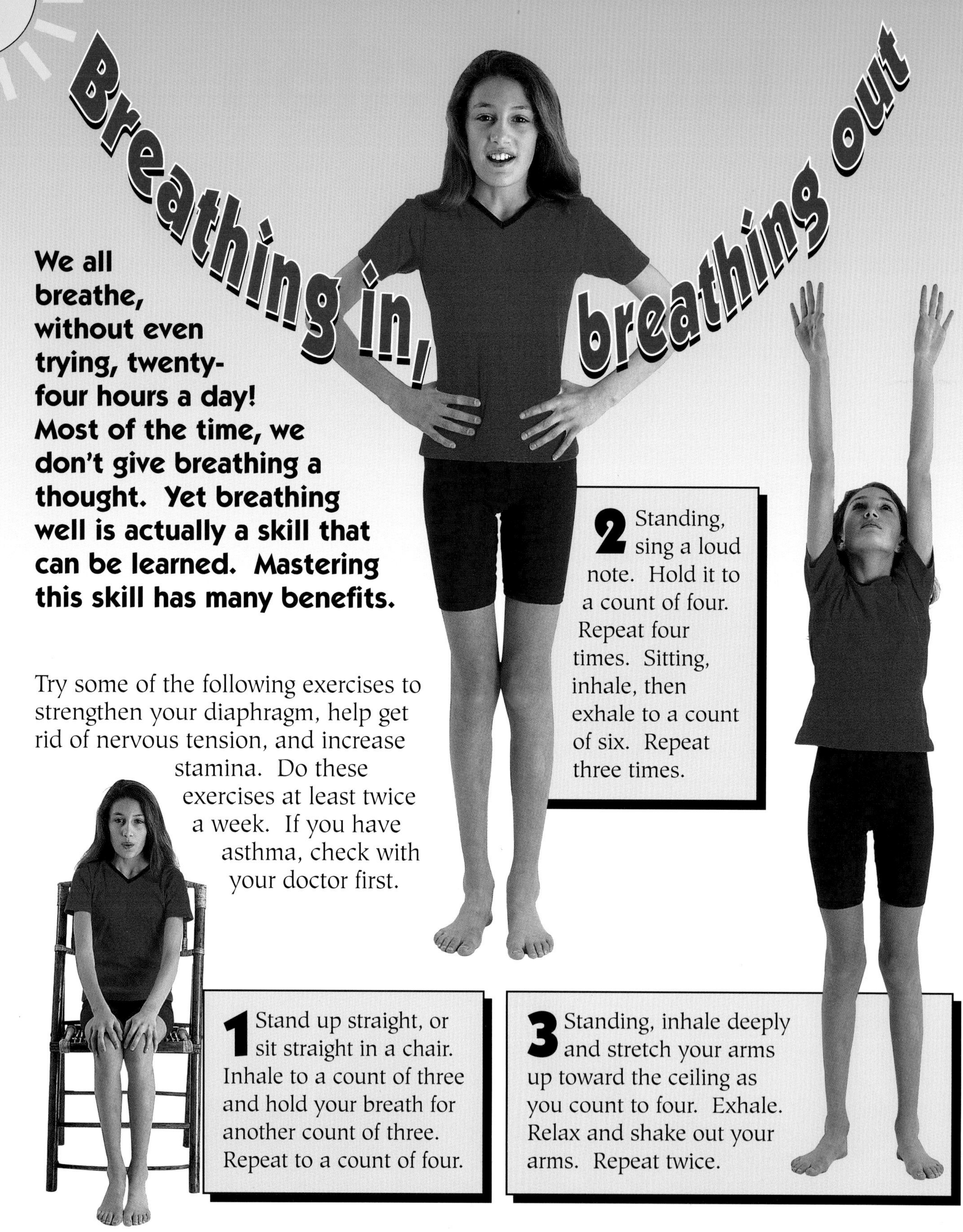

We all breathe, without even trying, twenty-four hours a day! Most of the time, we don't give breathing a thought. Yet breathing well is actually a skill that can be learned. Mastering this skill has many benefits.

Try some of the following exercises to strengthen your diaphragm, help get rid of nervous tension, and increase stamina. Do these exercises at least twice a week. If you have asthma, check with your doctor first.

1 Stand up straight, or sit straight in a chair. Inhale to a count of three and hold your breath for another count of three. Repeat to a count of four.

2 Standing, sing a loud note. Hold it to a count of four. Repeat four times. Sitting, inhale, then exhale to a count of six. Repeat three times.

3 Standing, inhale deeply and stretch your arms up toward the ceiling as you count to four. Exhale. Relax and shake out your arms. Repeat twice.

Q. WHY IS BREATHING DEEPLY IMPORTANT?

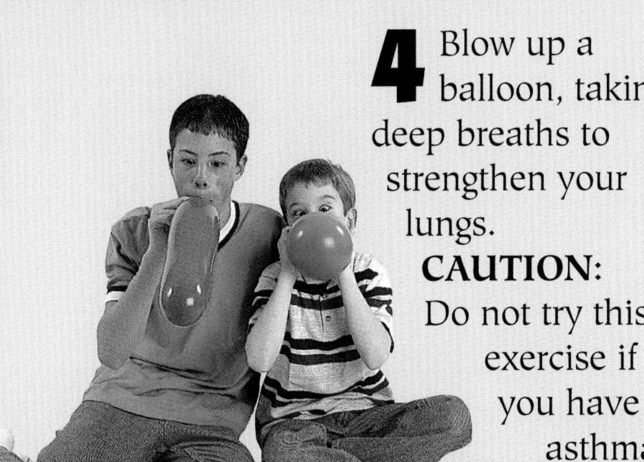

4 Blow up a balloon, taking deep breaths to strengthen your lungs.

CAUTION: Do not try this exercise if you have asthma.

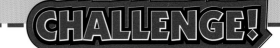

CHALLENGE!

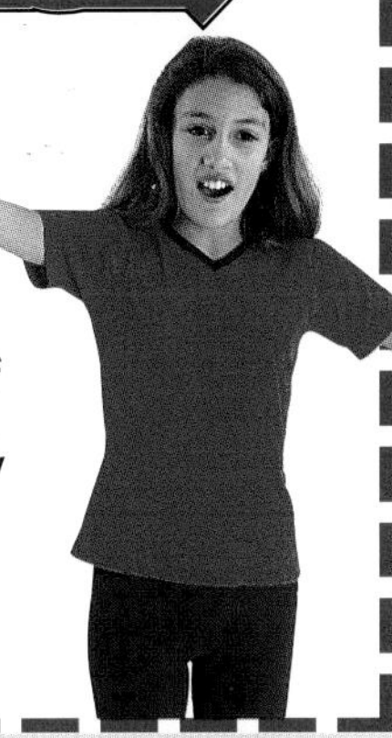

Pretend you are an opera star! Can you sing a loud note and hold it to a count of ten? Start by practicing to a count of five. Then hold the note longer, increasing the count by one number each day for five days. Bravo!

5 Standing, inhale. As you exhale, reach down toward your ankles. Don't stretch too hard; you don't have to touch your toes. Count to three. Inhale as you come back to an upright position.

7 Breathe deeply and slowly several times. When you're nervous — before an exam, perhaps — you might find yourself taking shallow breaths, using only the top of your rib cage. Breathe deeply to calm down.

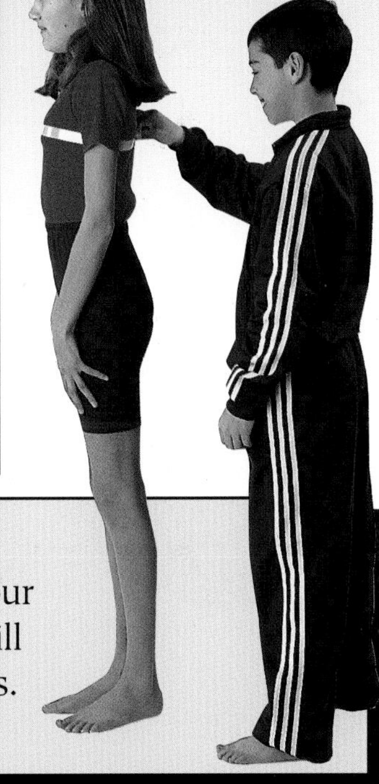

8 Have a friend hold some ribbon loosely around your chest. Inhale. The ribbon will tighten as your chest expands. Count to three. Exhale.

6 Lie down with your arms at your sides. Relax. Inhale slowly through your nose as you count to three. Exhale through your nose. Relax.

A. BREATHING DEEPLY CAN HELP YOU STAY CALM.

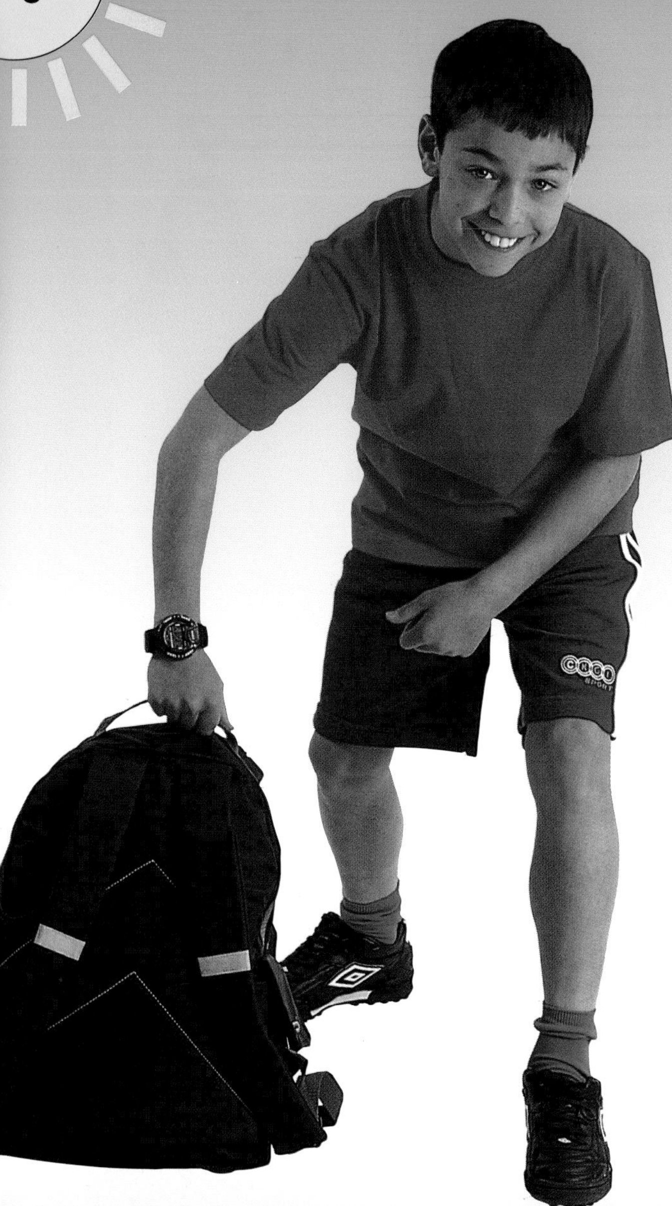

Stand tall,

Whatever your height, whatever your body shape, boy or girl, one thing is certain: you will always look your best if you have good posture. When you keep your back as straight as you can, good posture eventually becomes automatic.

Top models, film stars, and doctors agree: slouching just isn't pretty! Here are some golden rules that will help you look your most confident, fit, and attractive.

1 When you pick up something heavy, never — NEVER — bend at the waist to lift it. If you do, you could easily damage the muscles in your back. Always bend at the knees when you lift heavy things, and keep your back as straight as you can.

2 When you have to carry something heavy, for example, when you're helping with the grocery shopping, don't strain one side of your body by carrying everything in one hand. Balance the load. Put the groceries into two bags instead of one, and use both arms to carry them.

Q. WHY IS CARRYING A HEAVY SHOULDER BAG BAD FOR YOU?

sit up!

CHALLENGE!

Stand with your back against a wall and straighten your back, without forcing it too much, so a friend cannot easily put his or her arm behind you. Standing this straight might be difficult at first, but keep trying. This exercise will gradually help you straighten and strengthen your back, which will improve your posture.

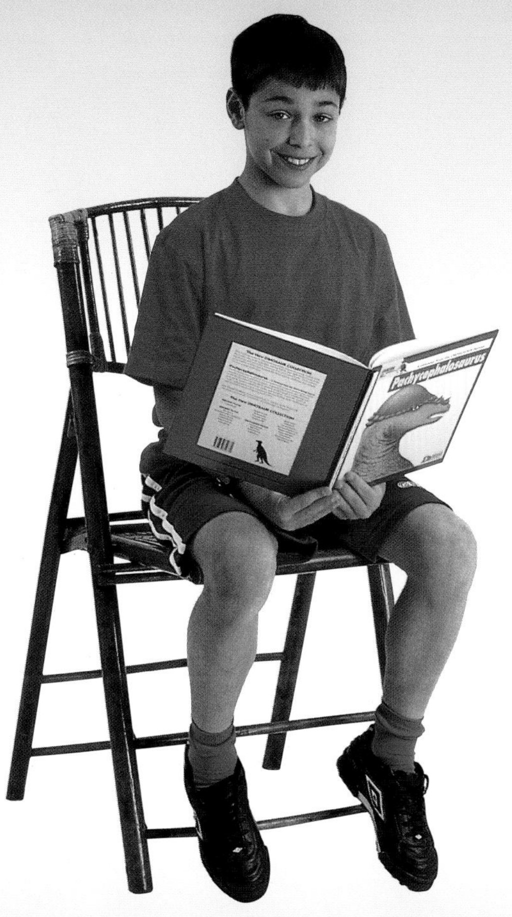

3 At school, it's always tempting to bend over your desk, hunching your back, when you are reading or writing or, at home, to slouch in a chair when you are watching TV. Sitting like this, however, can quickly make you round-shouldered. People who stand tall and sit straight against the back of a chair look more attractive and actually feel more comfortable. If you practice sitting properly, it should soon come naturally to you.

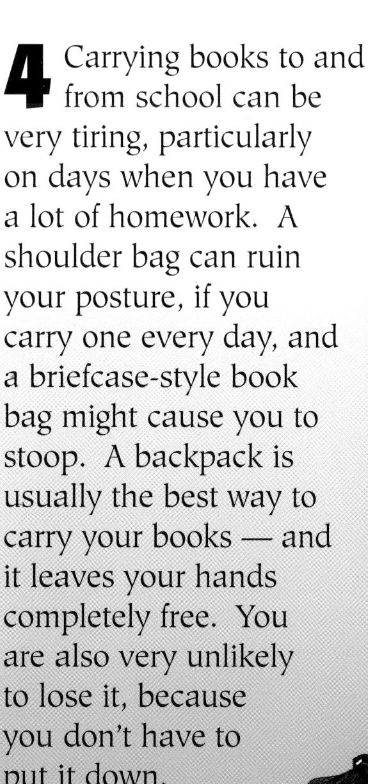

4 Carrying books to and from school can be very tiring, particularly on days when you have a lot of homework. A shoulder bag can ruin your posture, if you carry one every day, and a briefcase-style book bag might cause you to stoop. A backpack is usually the best way to carry your books — and it leaves your hands completely free. You are also very unlikely to lose it, because you don't have to put it down.

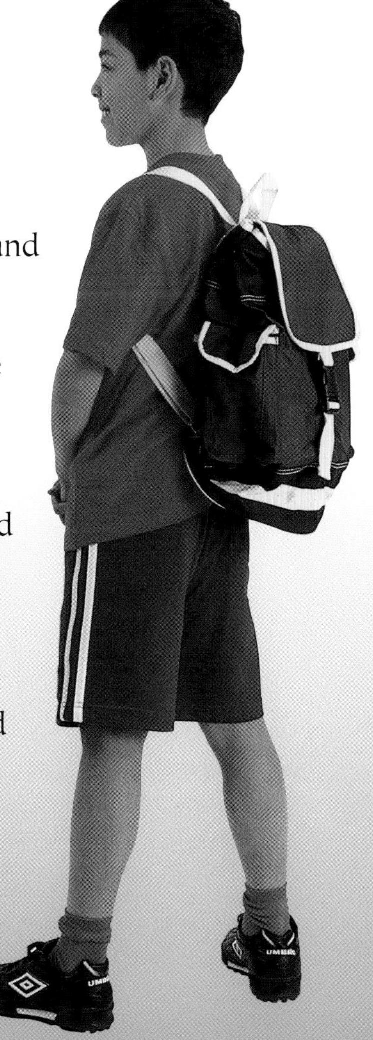

A. IT CAN RUIN YOUR POSTURE.

The funky five

A brief daily workout will not only help keep you flexible, it will also improve your circulation and lung function.

The following exercises can be done each day and should take only about five minutes. You don't need any equipment — just the desire to keep fit. Why not start your "funky five" program today?

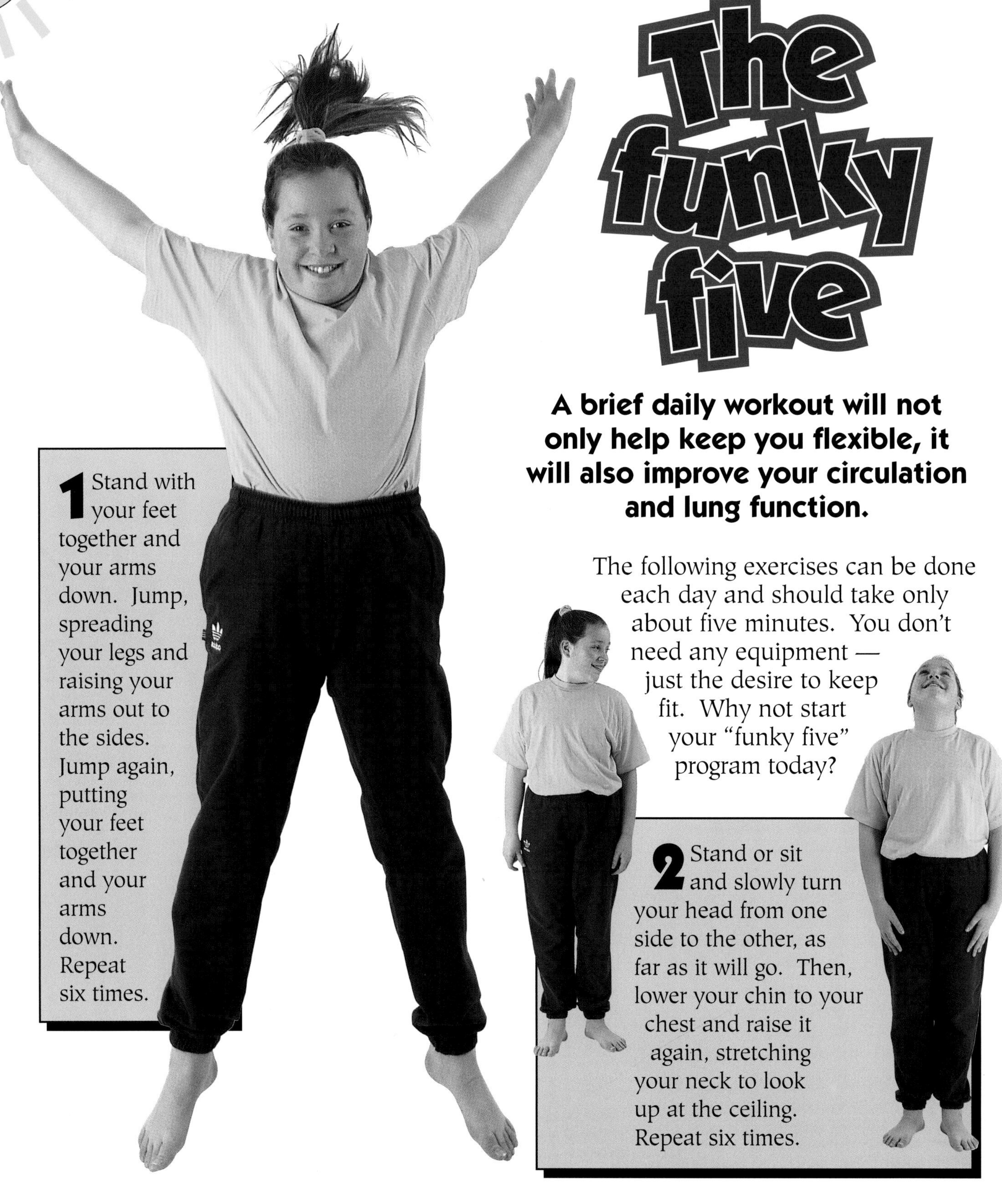

1 Stand with your feet together and your arms down. Jump, spreading your legs and raising your arms out to the sides. Jump again, putting your feet together and your arms down. Repeat six times.

2 Stand or sit and slowly turn your head from one side to the other, as far as it will go. Then, lower your chin to your chest and raise it again, stretching your neck to look up at the ceiling. Repeat six times.

Q. WHY IS EXERCISING DAILY GOOD FOR YOU?

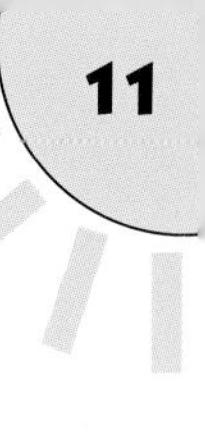

3 Sit on the floor with your legs stretched out and feet apart. Lean forward and try to touch your toes. Keep your back and legs straight. You might not be able to reach your toes at first, but keep trying to get a little closer each day. It won't matter if you never touch them.

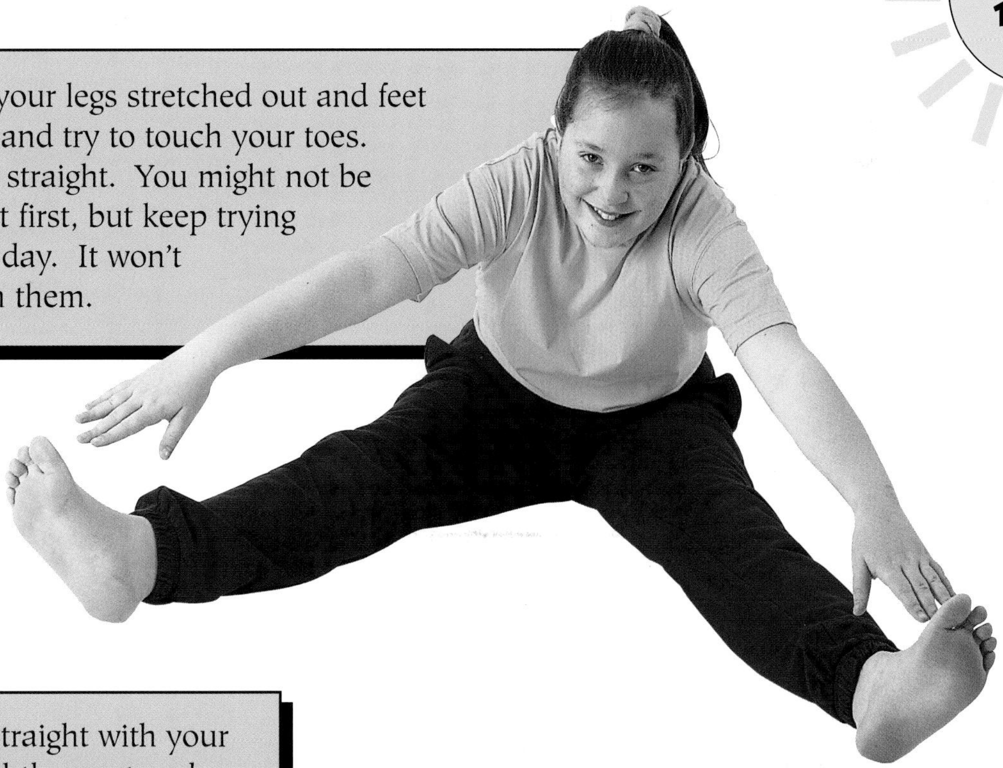

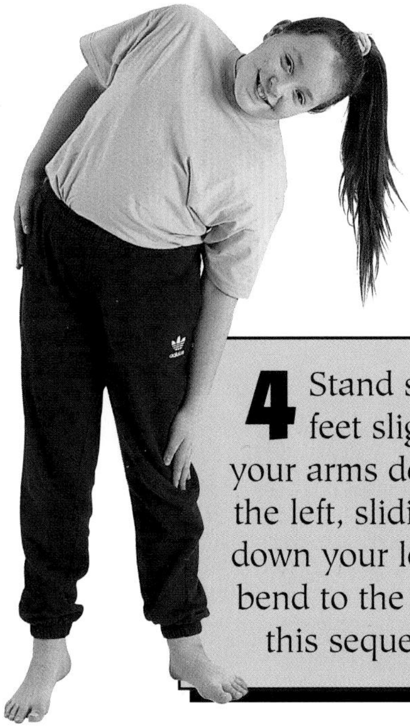

4 Stand straight with your feet slightly apart and your arms down. Bend to the left, sliding your left arm down your left leg. Then, bend to the right. Repeat this sequence six times.

CHALLENGE!

With one hand, hold a ruler over your shoulder. With your other hand, grasp the lower end of the ruler, as far up as possible (as shown). Each time you do this exercise, try to decrease the distance between your hands.

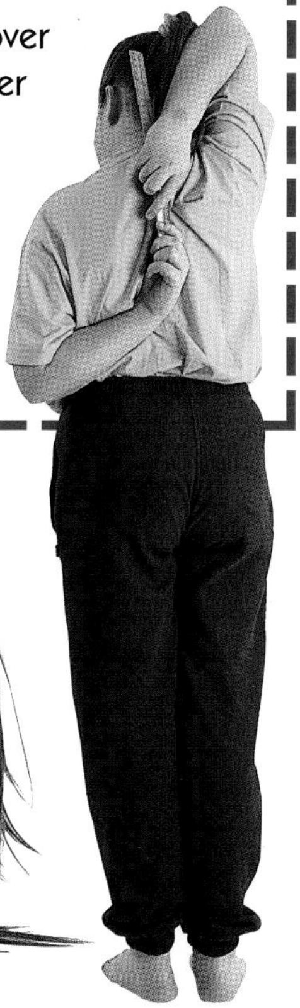

5 Lie down with your knees raised and your arms folded across your chest. Using only your stomach muscles — not your hands — try to sit up. It's difficult, isn't it? If you do this exercise twice a day, you should master it in a few weeks.

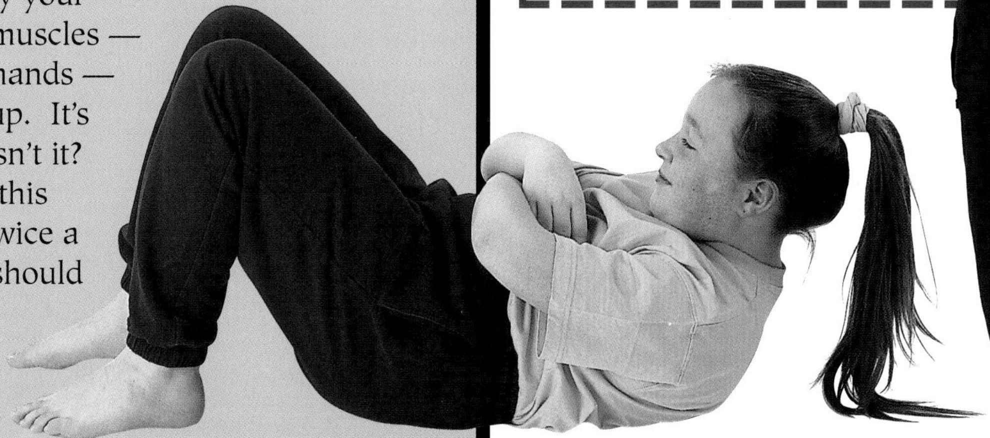

Working on a fitness program with a partner can keep you both on your toes, because you can each check that the other is exercising correctly.

Exercising

1 Lie down on your back, knees raised. Lift your head and shoulders off the floor. Count to three, then lie back down.

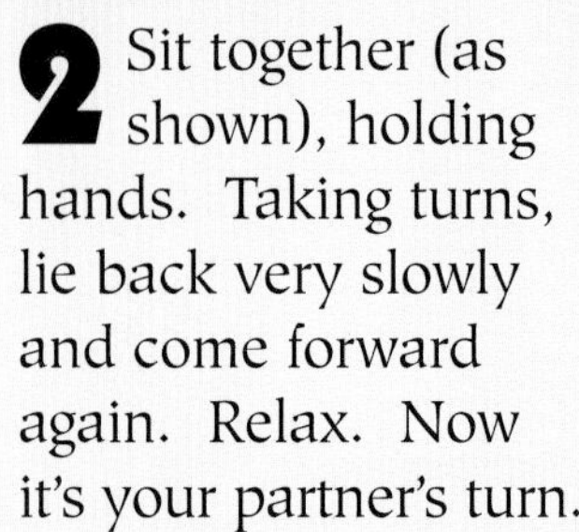

2 Sit together (as shown), holding hands. Taking turns, lie back very slowly and come forward again. Relax. Now it's your partner's turn.

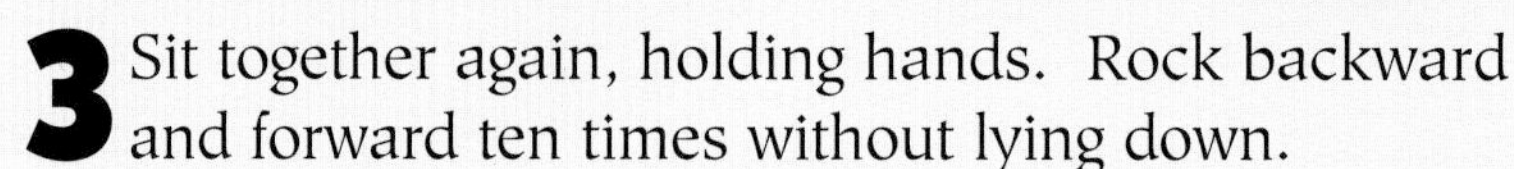

3 Sit together again, holding hands. Rock backward and forward ten times without lying down.

Q. WHY IS EXERCISING IN PAIRS A GOOD IDEA?

together

CHALLENGE!

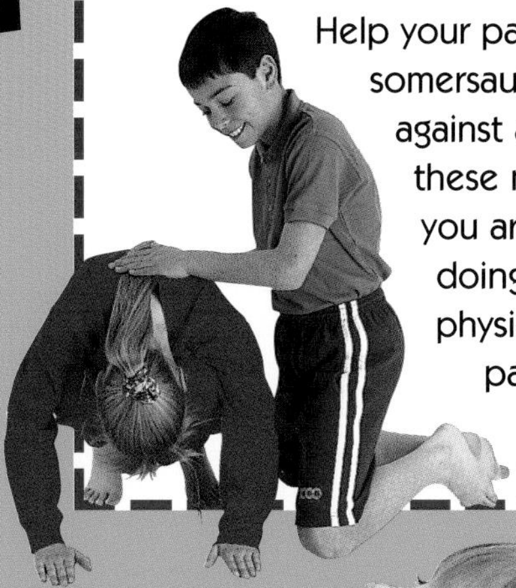

Help your partner try to do a somersault — or a handstand against a wall. Attempt these movements only if you are confident about doing them and are physically fit. Have your partner help you, too, if you want to try.

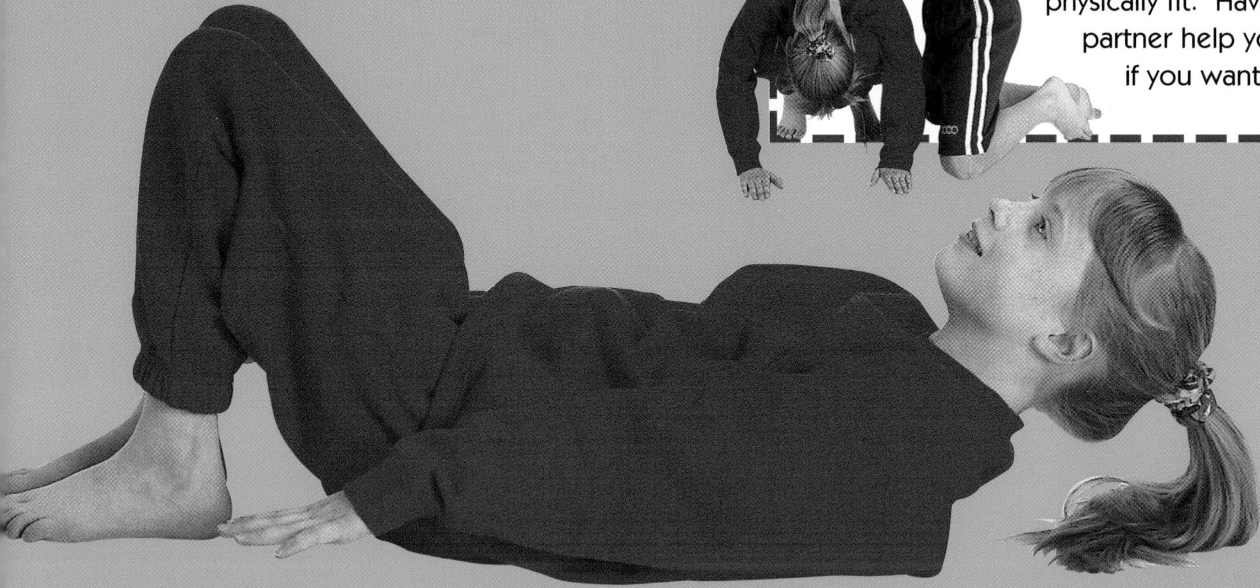

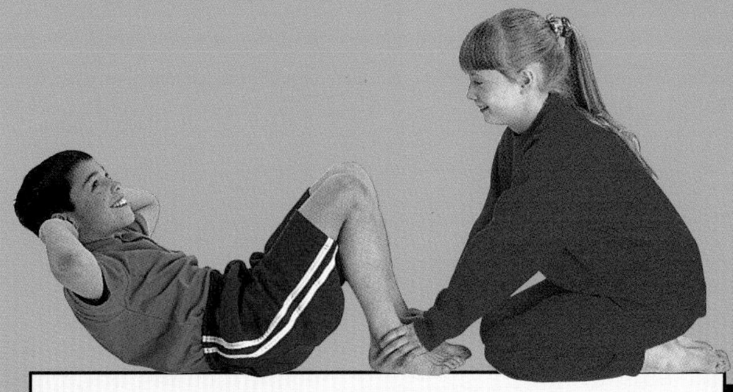

4 Lie on the floor, knees raised. Have your partner hold your feet down while you clasp your hands behind your head and raise your upper body off the floor. Change places so your partner can try.

5 Shadow-box by pretending to punch each other. This exercise is a good way to help you release any stored-up anger or frustration you have.

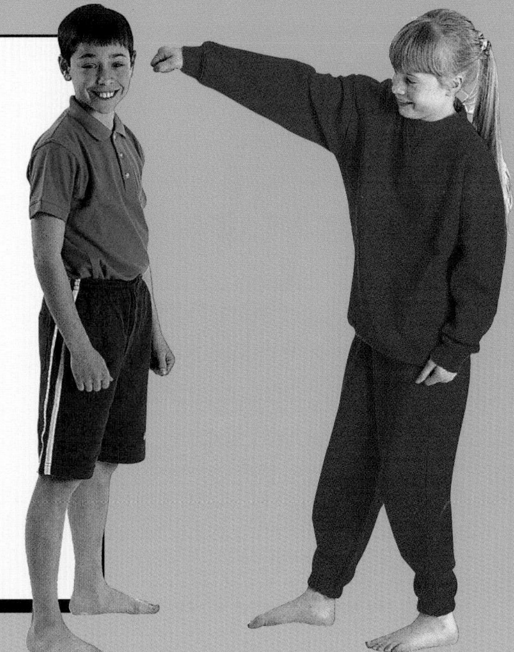

A. YOU CAN HELP EACH OTHER WITH THE EXERCISES.

TAKE A

You don't always have to stand up to exercise. Some fitness routines can be done sitting on a chair. Be sure to keep your back straight. A nice thing about chair exercising is almost anyone can do it — almost anywhere. These exercises are suitable even for someone who is older or someone not used to physical activity.

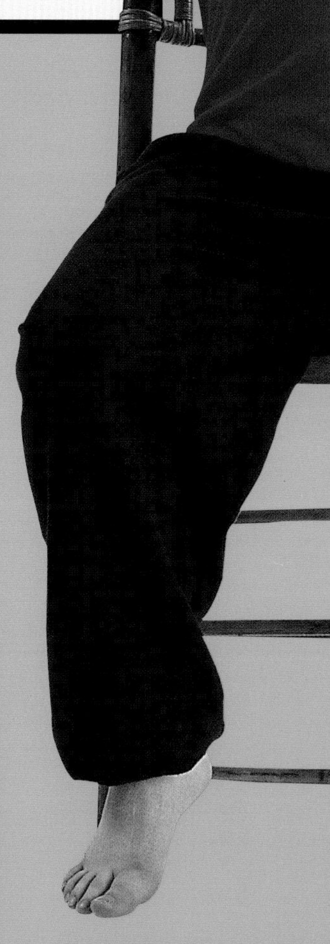

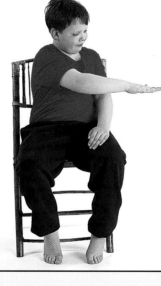

1 Lift both arms and stretch them out to the sides. Count to ten, then lower your arms again.

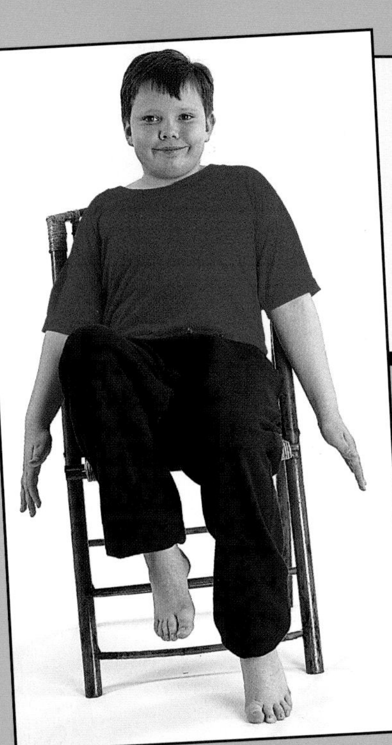

2 Raise one knee toward your chest, count to four, then lower it again. Repeat with the other knee.

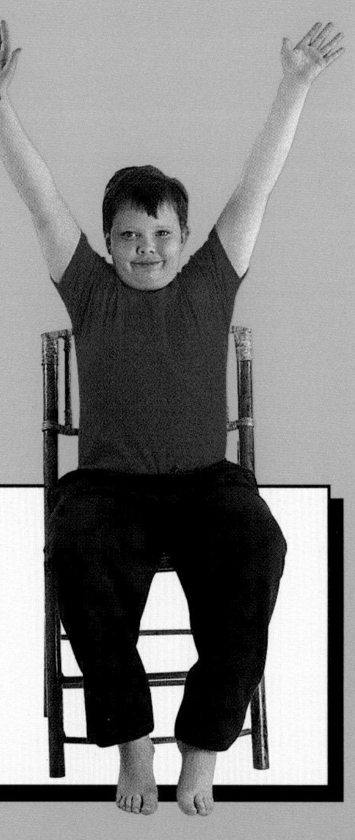

3 Sit up straight and raise both arms above your head. Count to four. Bring your arms down again.

4 Point with one arm across your body, looking toward your fingers (as shown). Bring that arm back and repeat with the other arm.

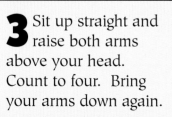

Q. WHO MIGHT WANT TO EXERCISE IN A CHAIR?

SEAT

CHALLENGE!

Sit in a chair and lean forward. Reach, as far as you can, toward your toes while still sitting in the chair. Stretch to a count of three. Then sit up straight.

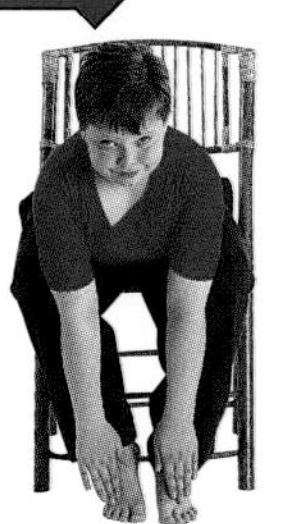

5 Stretch one leg out in front of you so that one foot is in the air while the other foot stays on the floor. Move the raised foot in a circle six times, first clockwise, then counterclockwise. Relax. Repeat with the other leg.

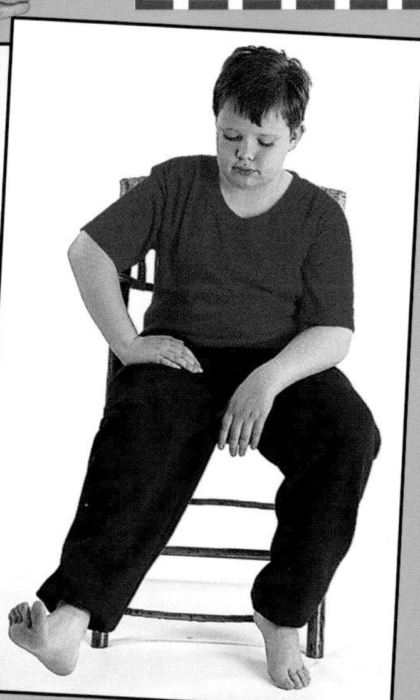

7 Sit up straight and clap your hands over your head four times in quick succession. Repeat.

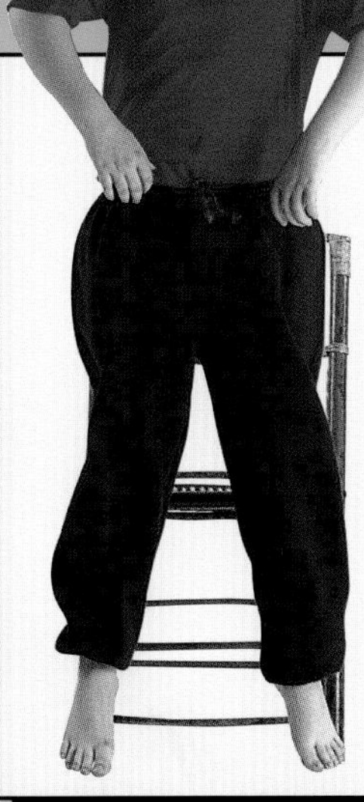

6 Sit up straight in a chair. Then, see how many times you can stand up and sit back down while someone counts out loud to twenty.

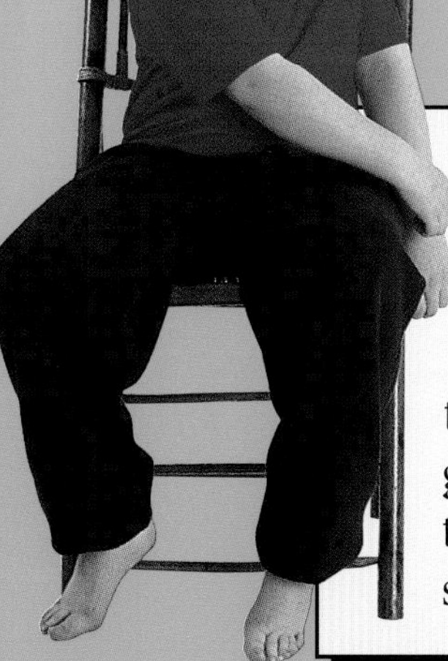

8 Sitting in a chair, twist the upper part of your body as far around to the right as it will go. Then twist to the left. Repeat this sequence four times.

A. ANYONE — ESPECIALLY THE DISABLED OR ELDERLY.

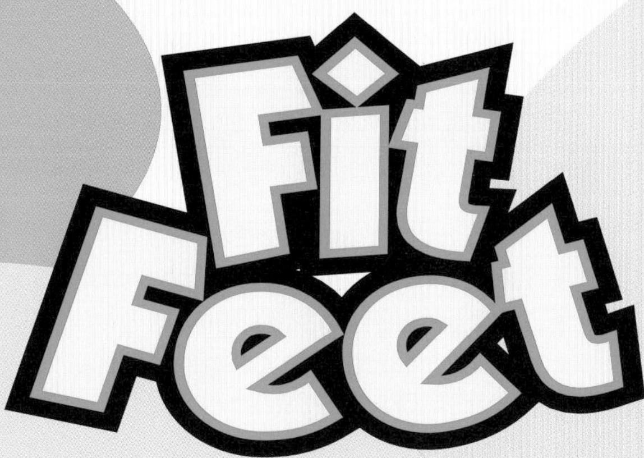

Fit Feet

Most of the time, your feet are confined in socks and shoes. Your toes, however, need freedom!

Exercising in bare feet is a good thing to do when you can do it safely — that is, when you have a clean, level, nonslip surface on which to work out.

You can do some specific exercises in bare feet to help keep them flexible and to build strong arches and straight toes. Try to do the following exercises, and the challenge, at least once a week — or whenever you have a little spare time.

1 Sit in a chair and, while counting to twenty, roll each foot, in turn, across a small rubber ball. Repeat four times.

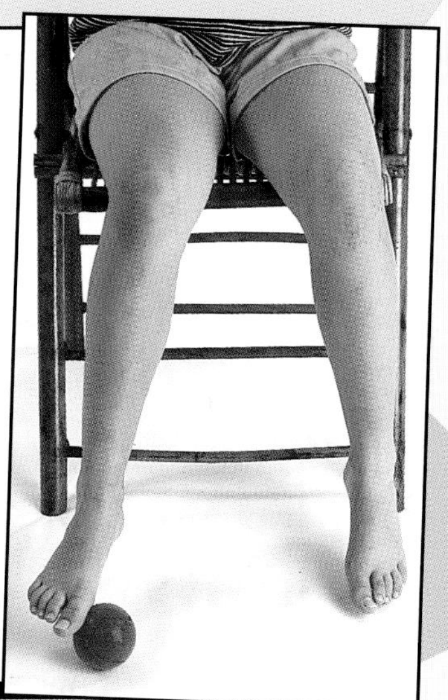

2 Sitting with feet flat on the floor, try to wiggle each toe one at a time. Do your toes obey? No one finds this exercise easy!

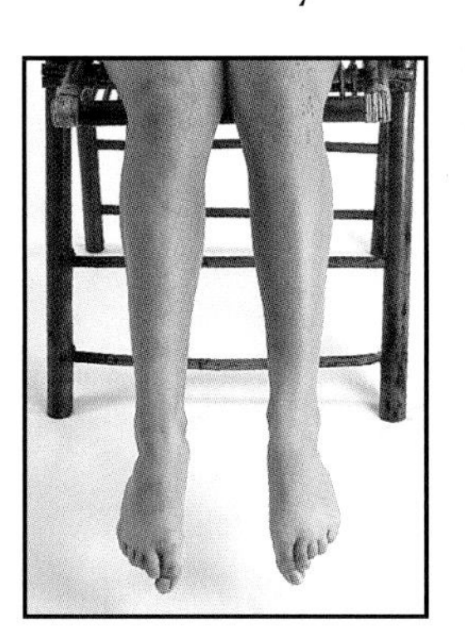

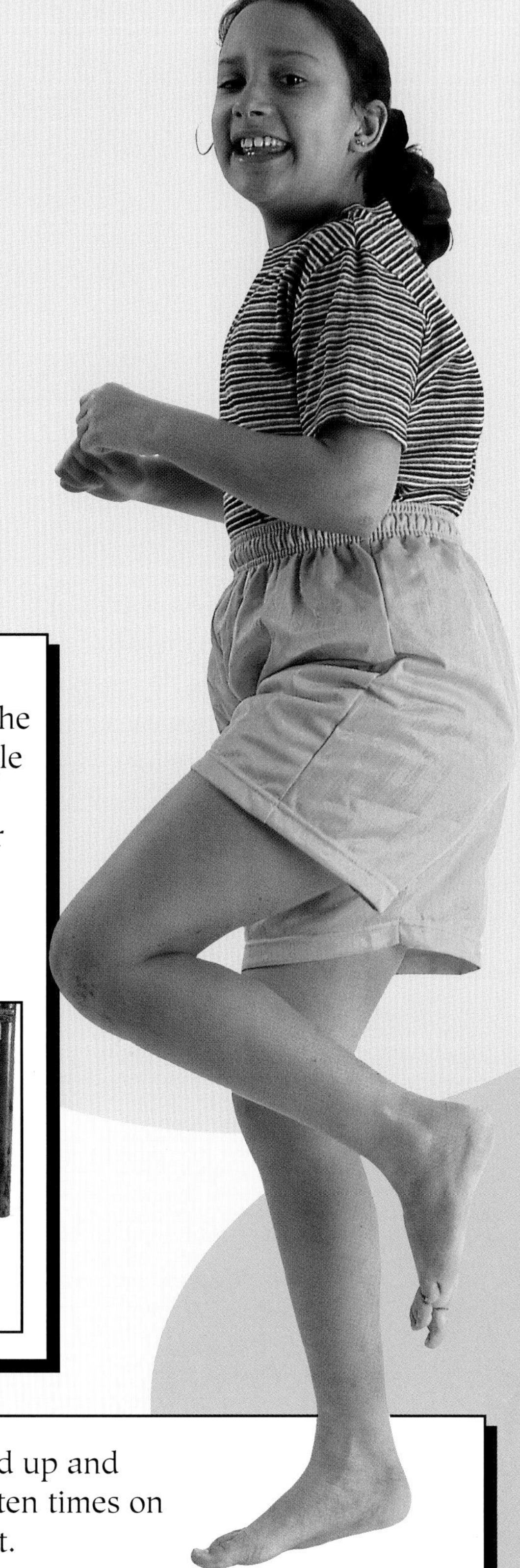

3 Stand up and hop ten times on each foot.

Q. WHY IS EXERCISING IN BARE FEET A GOOD THING TO DO?

4 Walk forward slowly on your toes, but not your tiptoes. Take ten steps, then turn and repeat. Now walk backward ten steps on your toes. (Don't bump into anything!) Turn and repeat.

5 With one foot, pick up a small beanbag between your toes and throw it as far as you can. Now try with the other foot. (If you don't have a beanbag, you can easily make one. Sew two square pieces of fabric together along three sides to form a bag. Fill the bag with beans, loosely, so it is not too stiff or solid. Sew up the fourth side.)

CHALLENGE!

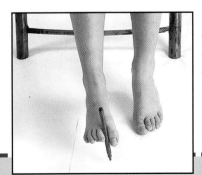

Place a piece of white paper on the floor in front of you. Hold a pencil between your big toe and the second toe of one foot. Try to write your name on the paper. You'll probably need days of practice to master this technique, but you'll have lots of fun trying — and your feet will be getting some good exercise!

A. IT STRENGTHENS YOUR ANKLES AND TOES.

Don't skip this!

Many athletes warm up before a game or sports event by jumping rope. You can, too!

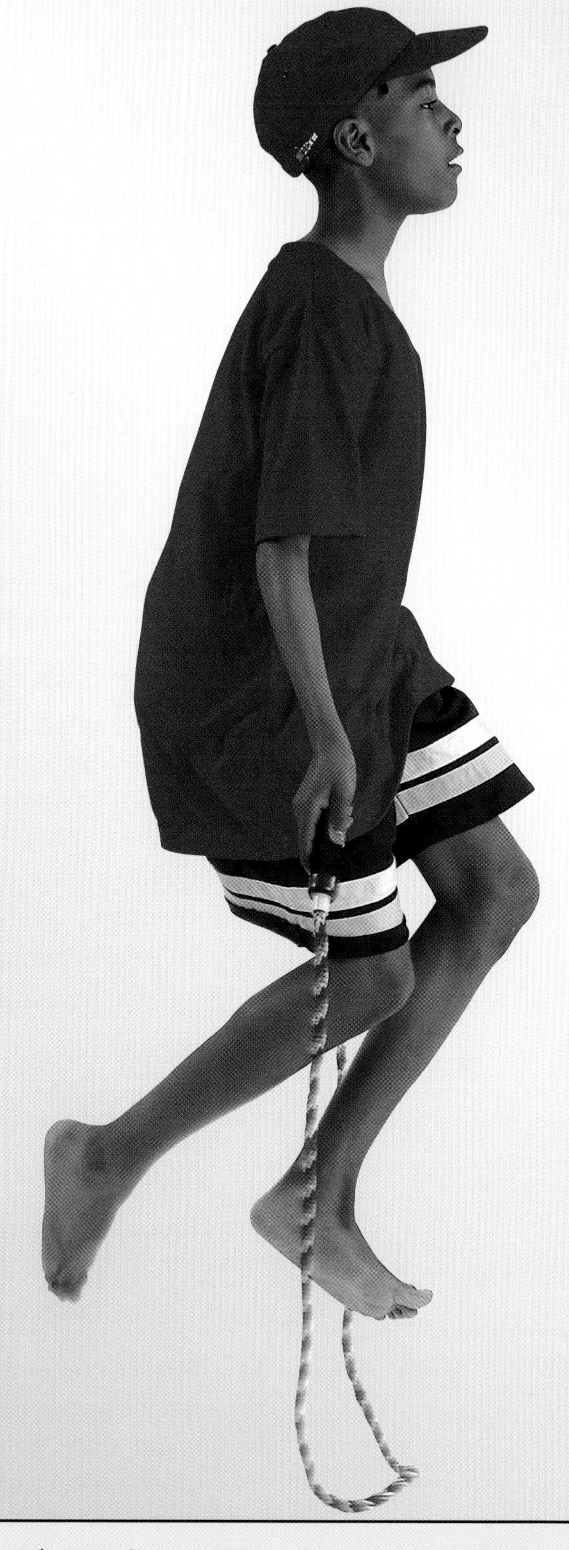

Jumping rope, as a playground game, has been popular throughout the world for centuries. Did you know, however, that a jump rope is a very useful and effective exercise tool and that jumping rope can improve both your circulation and your overall fitness?

Best of all, you can jump rope indoors or outdoors — and enjoy the weather when it's nice! When you jump indoors, make sure you have a nonslip surface to jump on and enough clear space in which to turn the rope. You will need the right length of rope for your height, too. If the rope is too long, it could trip you. So, jump right in! It doesn't take much time, and jumping to rhymes can make it even more fun.

1 Start by jumping the rope ten times without a break.

Q. WHY SHOULD YOU CHECK THE LENGTH OF YOUR JUMP ROPE?

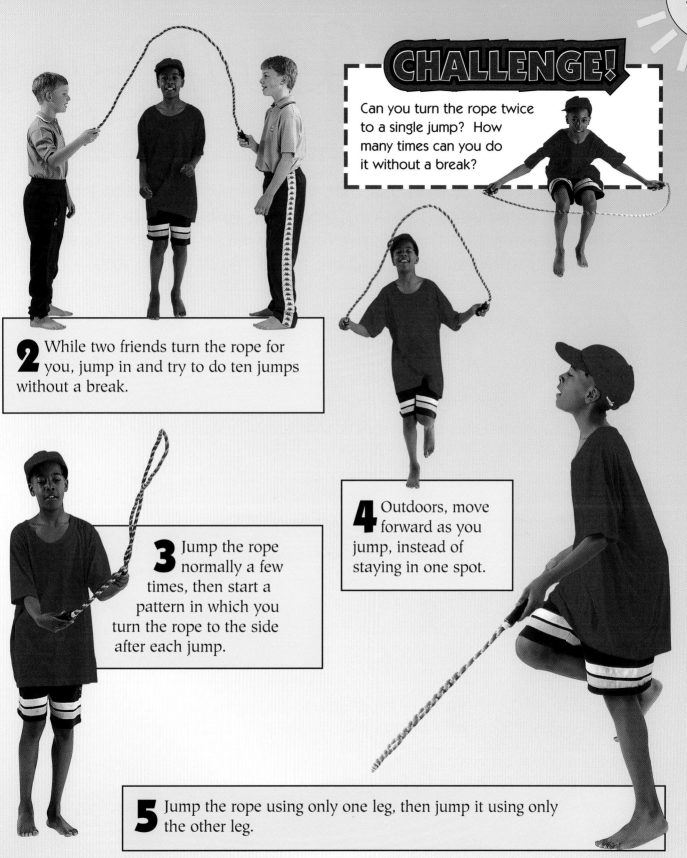

CHALLENGE!

Can you turn the rope twice to a single jump? How many times can you do it without a break?

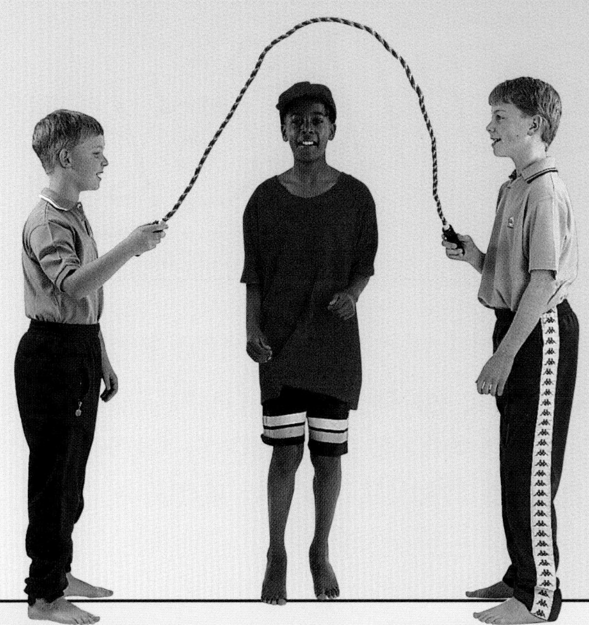

2 While two friends turn the rope for you, jump in and try to do ten jumps without a break.

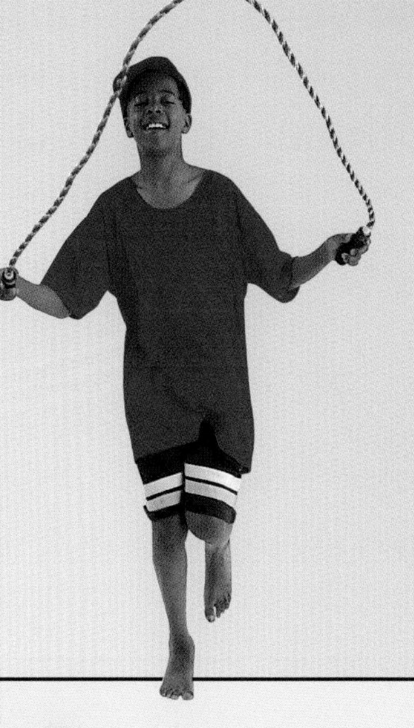

3 Jump the rope normally a few times, then start a pattern in which you turn the rope to the side after each jump.

4 Outdoors, move forward as you jump, instead of staying in one spot.

5 Jump the rope using only one leg, then jump it using only the other leg.

A. IF THE ROPE IS TOO LONG, YOU COULD TRIP ON IT.

Yoga for kids

Yoga is a form of exercise that started long ago in the East. To do some yoga positions, you have to be very flexible. The following positions, however, are simple postures, based on traditional yoga, and are not difficult to do well.

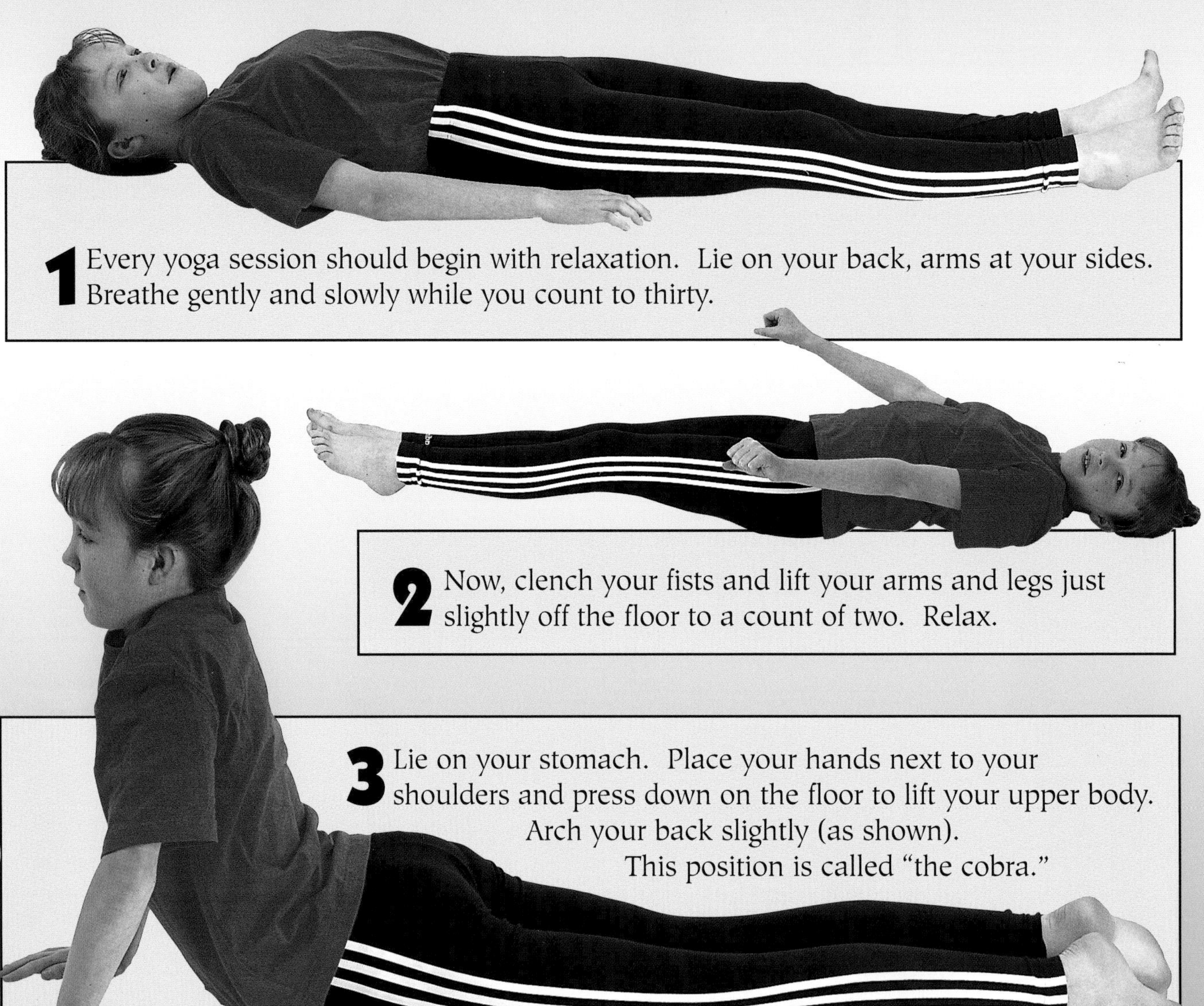

1 Every yoga session should begin with relaxation. Lie on your back, arms at your sides. Breathe gently and slowly while you count to thirty.

2 Now, clench your fists and lift your arms and legs just slightly off the floor to a count of two. Relax.

3 Lie on your stomach. Place your hands next to your shoulders and press down on the floor to lift your upper body. Arch your back slightly (as shown). This position is called "the cobra."

Q. HOW SHOULD EACH YOGA SESSION BEGIN?

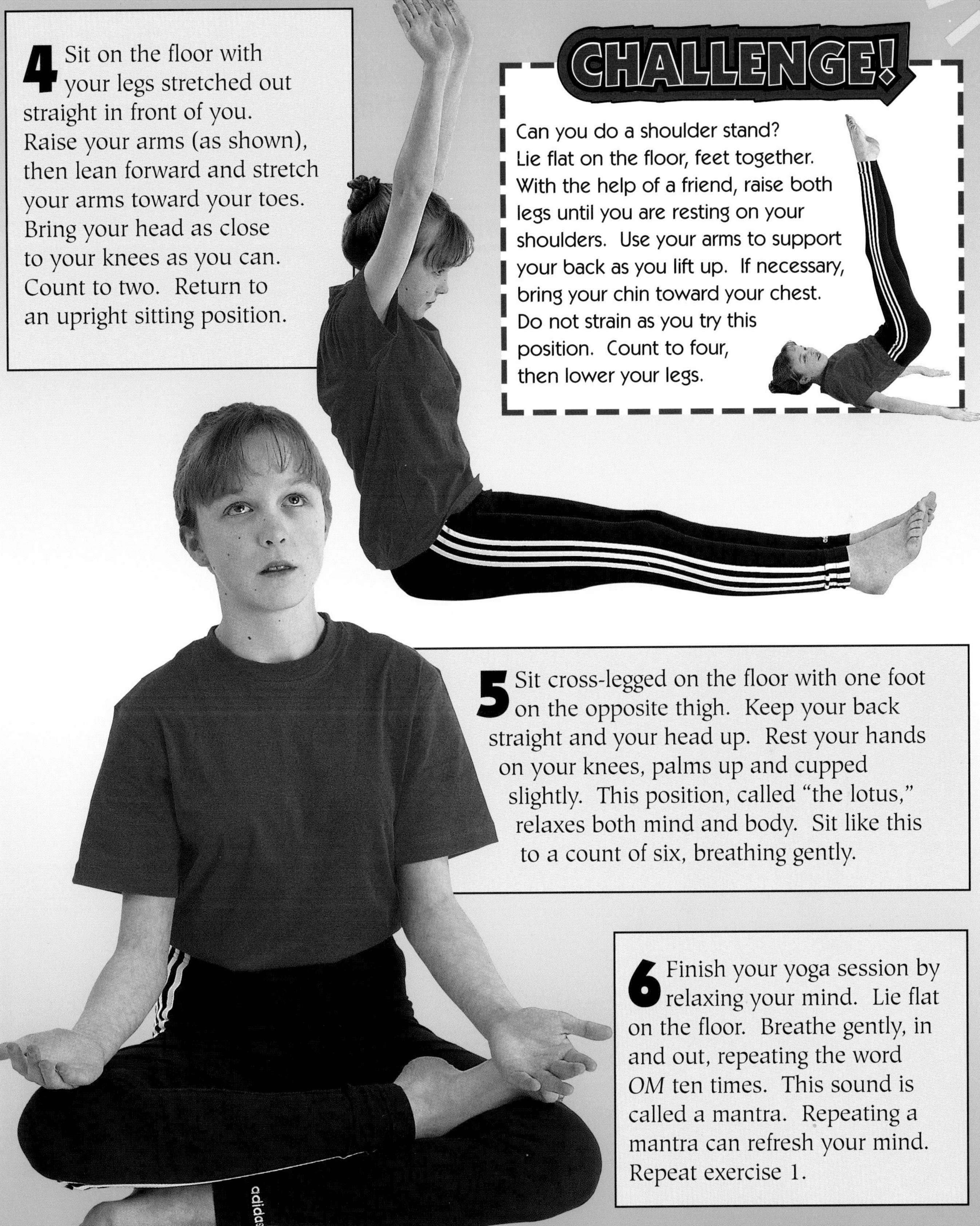

4 Sit on the floor with your legs stretched out straight in front of you. Raise your arms (as shown), then lean forward and stretch your arms toward your toes. Bring your head as close to your knees as you can. Count to two. Return to an upright sitting position.

CHALLENGE!

Can you do a shoulder stand? Lie flat on the floor, feet together. With the help of a friend, raise both legs until you are resting on your shoulders. Use your arms to support your back as you lift up. If necessary, bring your chin toward your chest. Do not strain as you try this position. Count to four, then lower your legs.

5 Sit cross-legged on the floor with one foot on the opposite thigh. Keep your back straight and your head up. Rest your hands on your knees, palms up and cupped slightly. This position, called "the lotus," relaxes both mind and body. Sit like this to a count of six, breathing gently.

6 Finish your yoga session by relaxing your mind. Lie flat on the floor. Breathe gently, in and out, repeating the word *OM* ten times. This sound is called a mantra. Repeating a mantra can refresh your mind. Repeat exercise 1.

A. EACH YOGA SESSION SHOULD BEGIN WITH A RELAXATION EXERCISE.

Animal antics

These exercises have a wildlife theme and are based on the characteristics of several different creatures. When you do them, try to pretend you really are the animal. Exercise doesn't have to be boring!

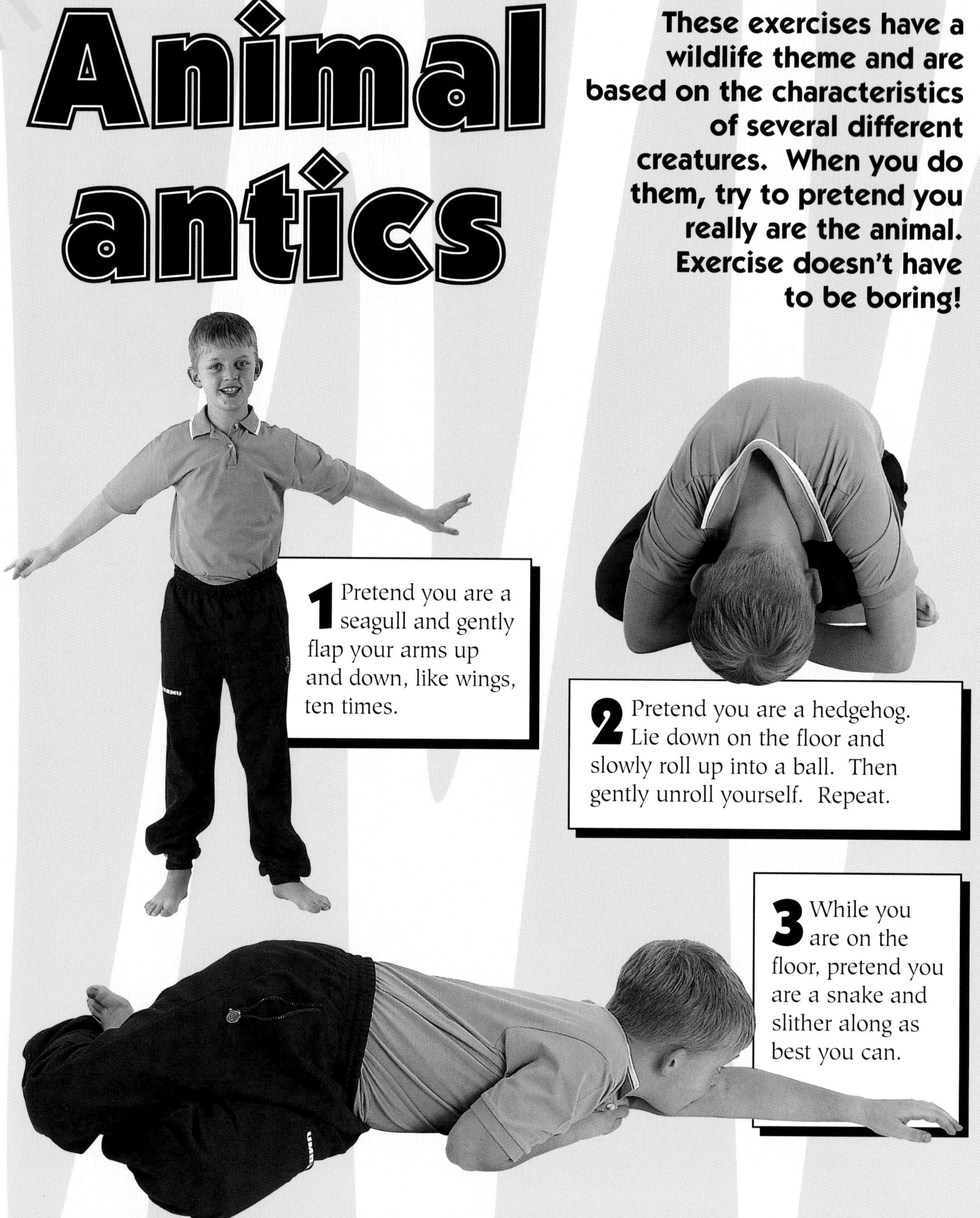

1 Pretend you are a seagull and gently flap your arms up and down, like wings, ten times.

2 Pretend you are a hedgehog. Lie down on the floor and slowly roll up into a ball. Then gently unroll yourself. Repeat.

3 While you are on the floor, pretend you are a snake and slither along as best you can.

Q. WHICH PARTS OF YOUR BODY WILL A FROG EXERCISE STRENGTHEN?

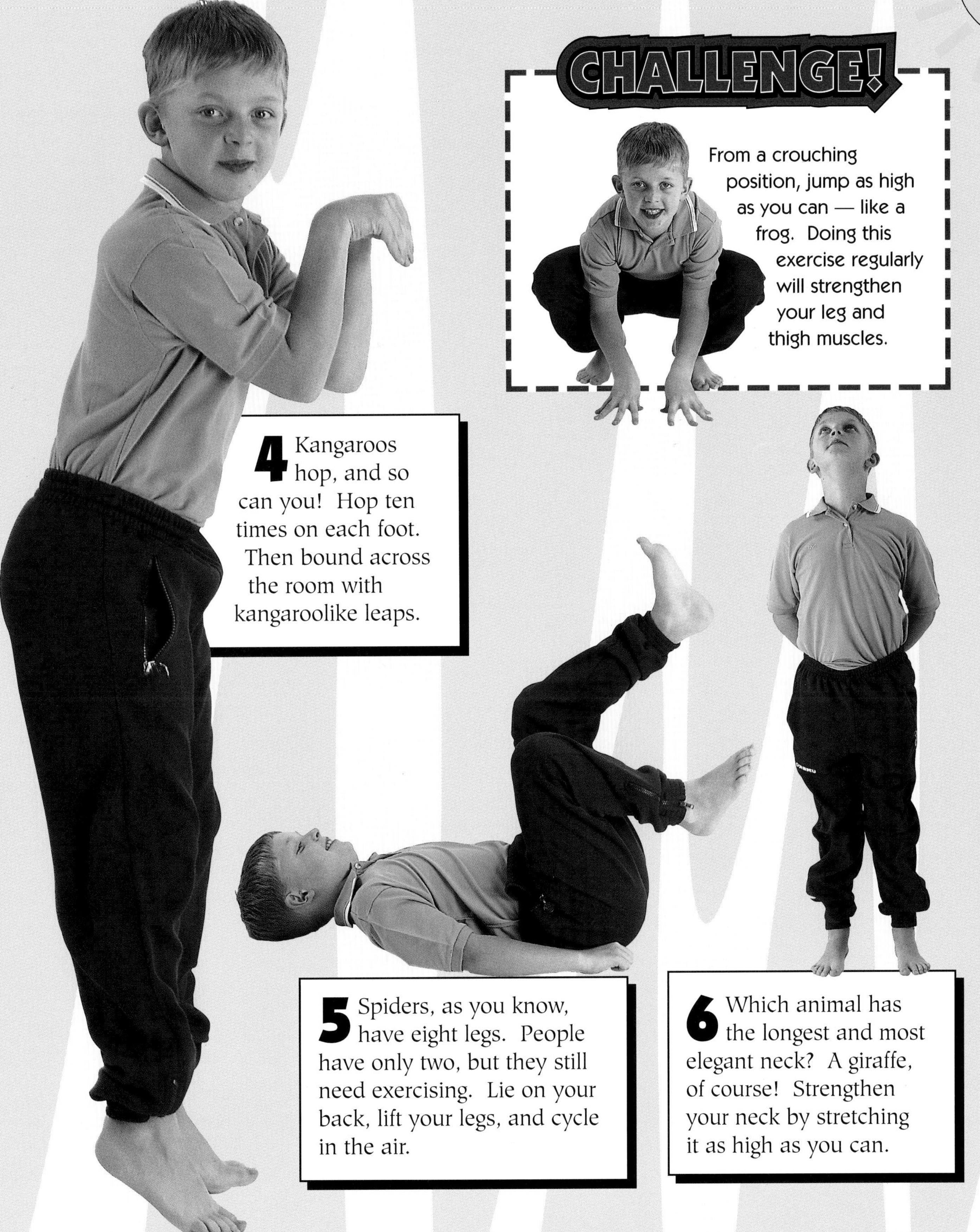

CHALLENGE!

From a crouching position, jump as high as you can — like a frog. Doing this exercise regularly will strengthen your leg and thigh muscles.

4 Kangaroos hop, and so can you! Hop ten times on each foot. Then bound across the room with kangaroolike leaps.

5 Spiders, as you know, have eight legs. People have only two, but they still need exercising. Lie on your back, lift your legs, and cycle in the air.

6 Which animal has the longest and most elegant neck? A giraffe, of course! Strengthen your neck by stretching it as high as you can.

A. A FROG EXERCISE STRENGTHENS YOUR LEGS AND THIGHS.

Dancercise

Exercising to music is a lot of fun — by yourself, with a partner, or in a group.

Moving in time to any kind of music adds rhythm to your exercise routine and livens up the action. Choose slow music if you want to exercise in a relaxed way, and faster music if you feel like doing something more energetic and working up a sweat. You can try doing several of the exercise routines in this book to music.

You probably have come across the word *aerobics* in connection with exercise. It simply means "with air." In aerobic dance sessions, the exercise is vigorous to increase the amount of oxygen that reaches your muscles. Aerobic dance strengthens lung function and builds stamina. Be careful, however, not to overdo. Stop as soon as you are out of breath.

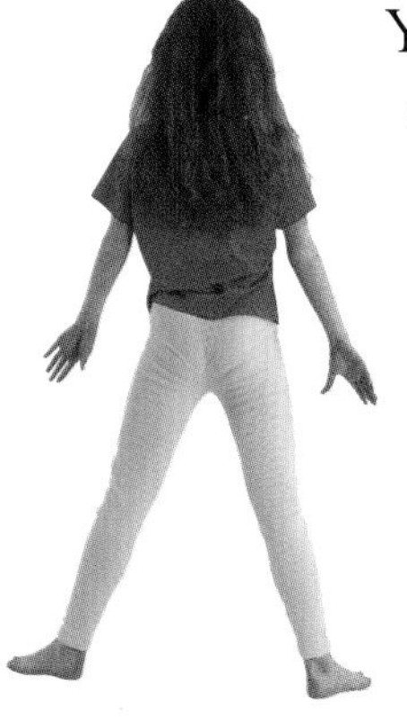

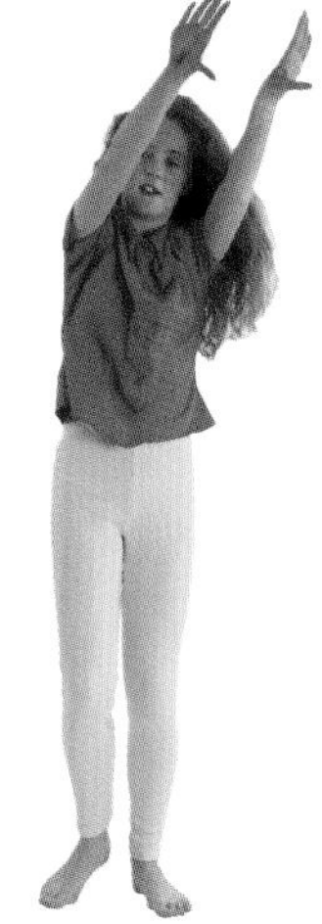

Dancing is good for you — physically, mentally, and socially. When you dancercise, feel free to make up your own steps. Wear loose clothing and light shoes — or dance in bare feet on

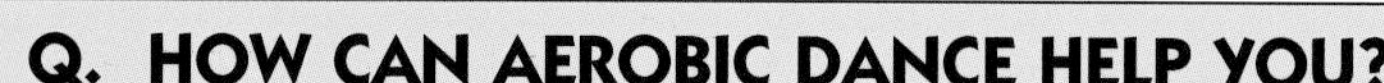

Q. HOW CAN AEROBIC DANCE HELP YOU?

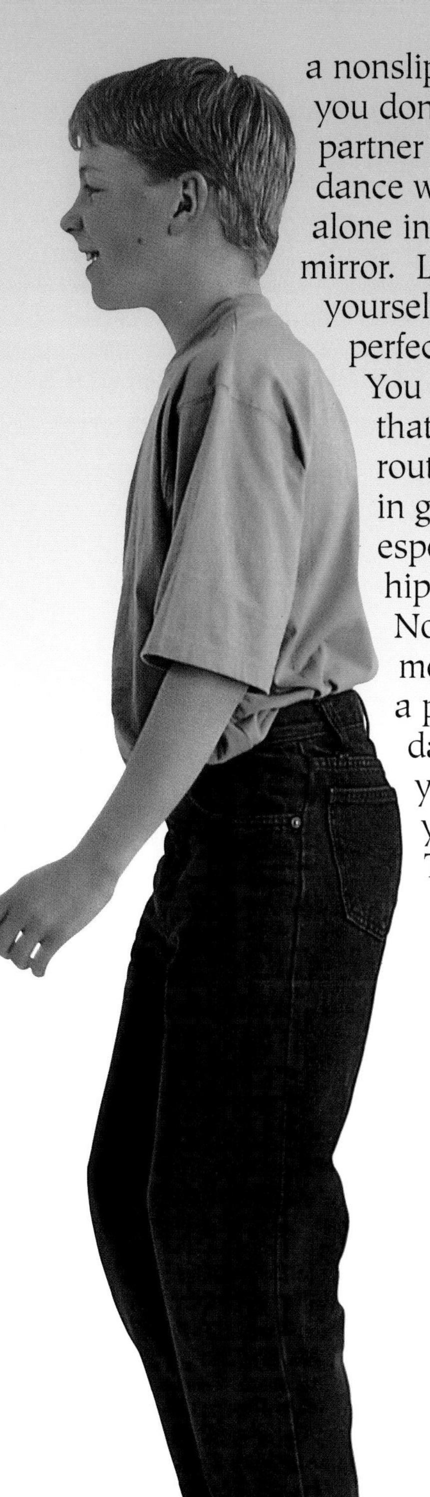

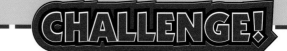

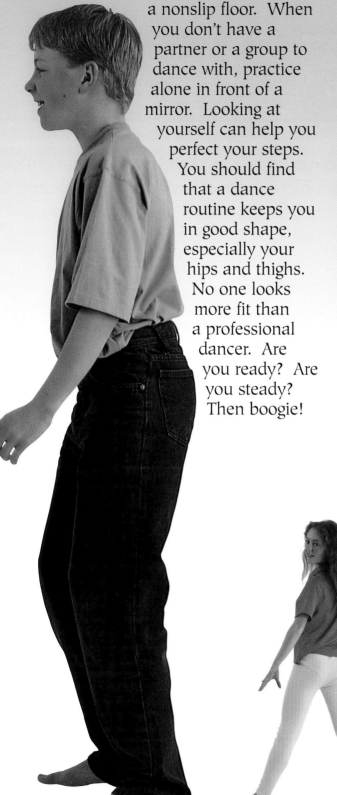

a nonslip floor. When you don't have a partner or a group to dance with, practice alone in front of a mirror. Looking at yourself can help you perfect your steps. You should find that a dance routine keeps you in good shape, especially your hips and thighs. No one looks more fit than a professional dancer. Are you ready? Are you steady? Then boogie!

CHALLENGE!

Play some music (reggae might be good for this routine). Have two friends hold a rope at just above the height of your waist. Move forward, bending slightly backward, and try to pass under the rope (as shown). This dance is known as the "limbo." It comes from the West Indies. Be careful not to strain when you try it. If any part of you starts to hurt, stop dancing immediately. You have to be very flexible to meet this challenge, but practice will help.

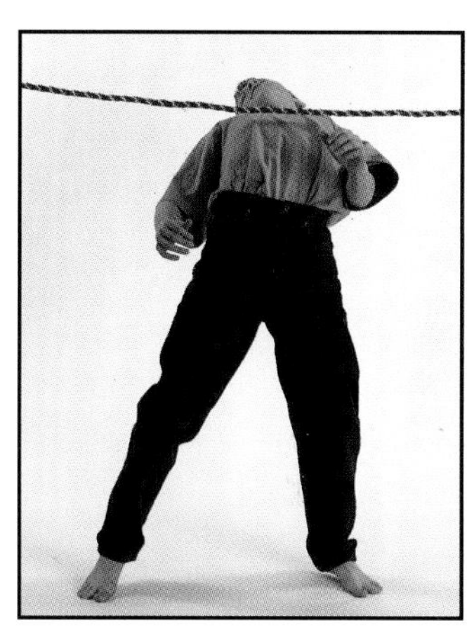

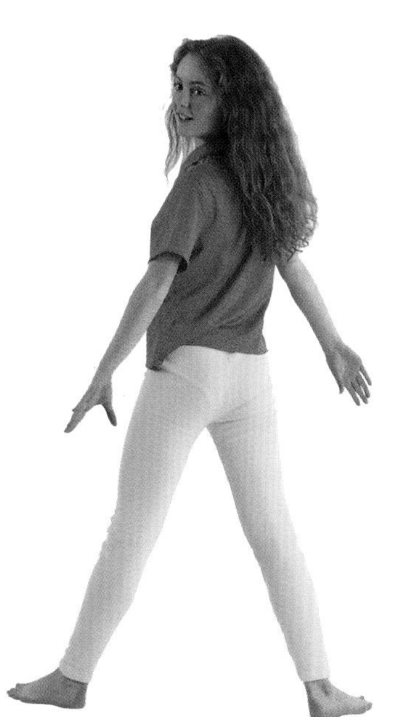

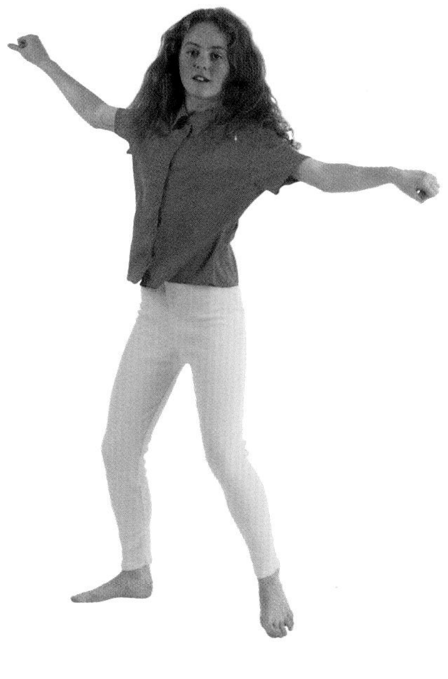

A. AEROBIC DANCE CAN BUILD STAMINA.

Jogging along

Jogging is one of the best exercises to improve stamina. For safety's sake, jog with a group of friends or where lots of people are around. Jog on grass — it's better for your feet than a hard sidewalk — and avoid harmful exhaust fumes by not jogging too close to traffic.

Here are some tips to help you jog as comfortably and healthfully as possible.

1 Wear shoes that are designed for running, and be sure the laces are tied securely so you don't trip on them. Shoes with cushioned soles are best. Avoid tight clothing. Depending on the weather, wear comfortable shorts or a warm-up suit when you jog.

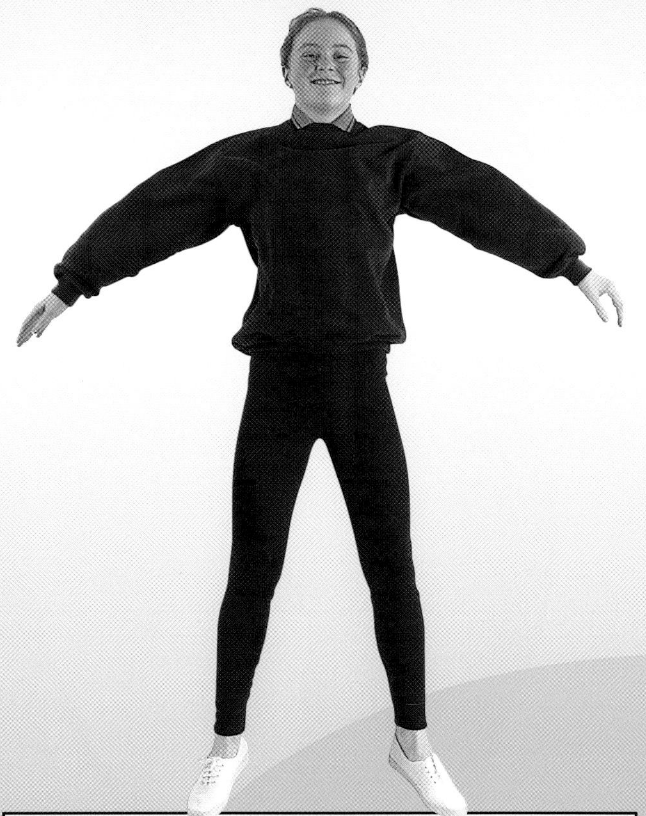

2 Do a few warm-up exercises, such as jumping jacks or running in place, before you start jogging.

Q. WHY CAN JOGGING ALONG A MAIN ROAD BE BAD FOR YOU?

CHALLENGE!

Can you talk to your running partners while you jog? If not, you probably are jogging too fast. Slow down, until you are able to speak easily, and always maintain a steady rhythm.

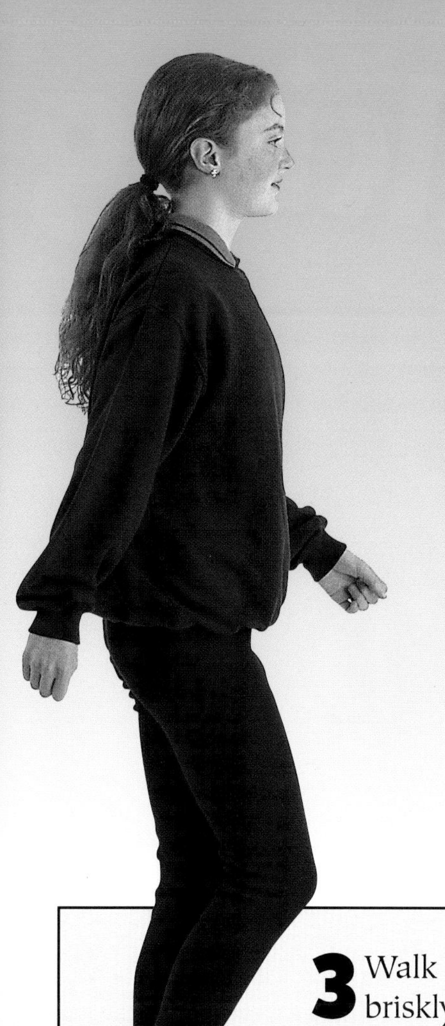

3 Walk briskly for about a minute, then start to jog. Never jog quickly. Speed is not important; a slow pace is best. If you run out of breath, stop jogging. When you first start a jogging program, jog for only about three minutes a day. After a week or so, increase your time by one minute per day. Work your way up to a six-minute maximum.

4 Experienced joggers recommend that you do not lift your legs too high as you jog, and suggest that you might enjoy listening to music while jogging.

5 When you jog, keep your body as straight as possible. Breathe easily and rhythmically through your mouth, rather than through your nose.

A. THE TRAFFIC CAN BE DANGEROUS, AND THE EXHAUST FUMES CAN BE HARMFUL.

Making

You don't have to be strikingly beautiful or extraordinarily handsome to attract others. An interesting and lively face is just as appealing. Exercise can help!

You have many muscles in your jaws, throat, and neck that will benefit from being strengthened. Stand or sit in front of a mirror and have fun "making faces" with the following exercises. The young people in these photographs seem to be enjoying the routine enormously! Do these exercises twice a week, for just a few minutes. They will also improve your circulation.

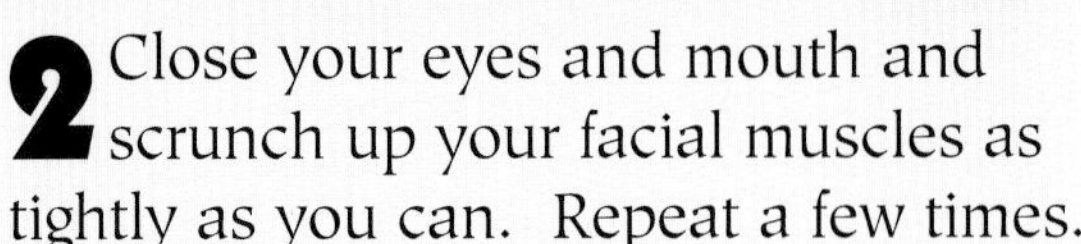

2 Close your eyes and mouth and scrunch up your facial muscles as tightly as you can. Repeat a few times.

1 Watch your reflection and purse your lips (as shown). Say the word "BOO!" as loudly as you can. Repeat six times.

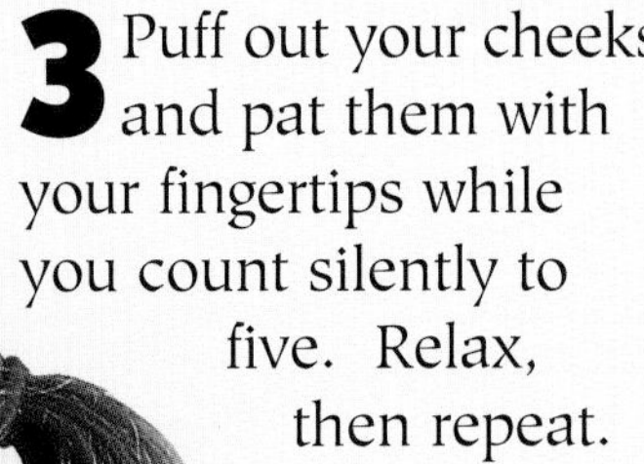

3 Puff out your cheeks and pat them with your fingertips while you count silently to five. Relax, then repeat.

Q. WHY IS EXERCISING YOUR NECK A GOOD THING TO DO?

faces

CHALLENGE!

Try to wrinkle your nose. You'll probably find it hard to do, at first, but it becomes easier with practice. Some people can even wiggle their ears!

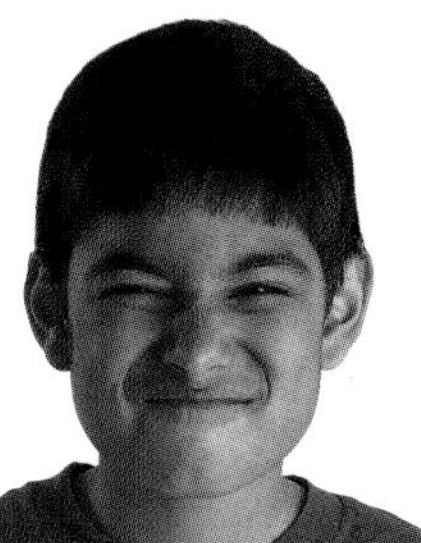

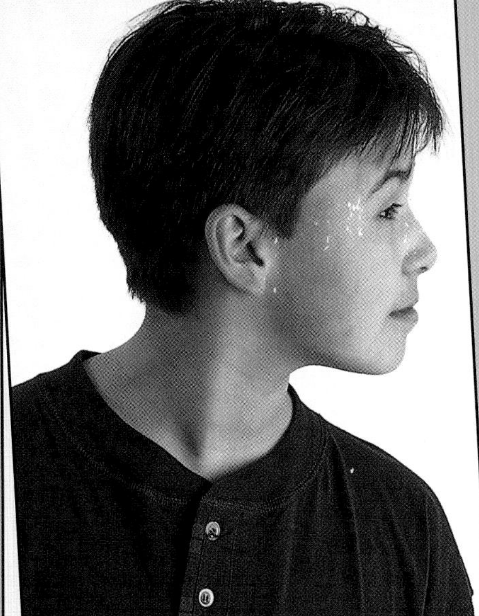

4 Turn your head to the right and look over your shoulder. Repeat this exercise, turning to the left.

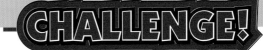

5 Lift your neck up as far as possible and roll your head around clockwise. Repeat, going counterclockwise.

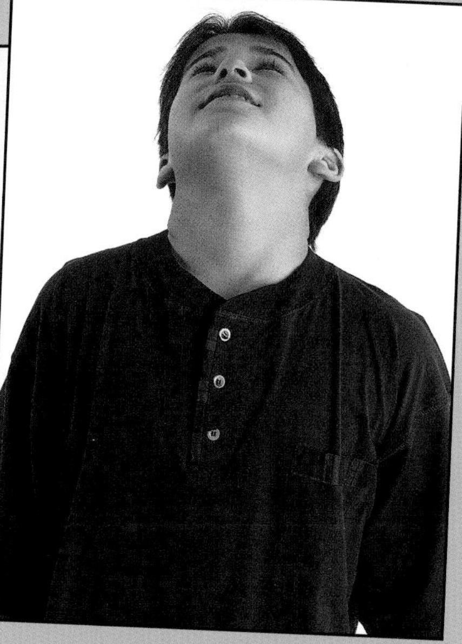

6 Open your eyes and mouth as widely as you can, then shout or sing out loudly. Repeat.

A. A FLEXIBLE NECK WILL IMPROVE YOUR POSTURE AND SPORTS PERFORMANCE.

Glossary

aerobics — a type of exercise, such as running or swimming, that improves breathing and circulation by helping the body take in more oxygen.

asthma — an illness, often caused by allergies, that causes attacks of coughing, wheezing, and gasping for air.

circulation — the movement of blood pumped by the heart through veins and arteries in the body.

clasp — (v) to hold firmly in your hands or arms; to grip or grasp.

clench — to close and press tightly together, such as making a fist.

confined — kept inside, usually in a closed-up area without much space.

crouch — to lower the body close to the ground mainly by bending at the knees and the hips.

diaphragm — a muscular wall that separates the chest and the abdomen in a person's body, and in the bodies of most other mammals.

expand — to get bigger or wider; to open up or unfold.

fitness — the condition of being in good physical health.

flexible — able to move and bend easily without breaking.

frustration — a feeling of defeat or discouragement over not being able to do or have something you want.

function — (n) the activity that someone or something is designed for or equipped to do; the purpose of something.

hedgehog — a small mammal in Africa, Asia, or Europe that, like a porcupine, has spines on its back to protect it but also rolls itself into a ball, making the spines stick straight out.

master — (v) to do something very well, like an expert.

posture — the way a person holds his or her body, especially while standing or sitting.

reggae — a type of music that combines a native Jamaican style with today's rock and soul rhythms.

routine — a series of actions that are repeated again and again.

slither — to slide smoothly along a surface, like a snake.

slouch — to sit, stand, or walk with a rounded back and drooping shoulders.

stamina — strength to keep going for a long time, especially to keep going until something ends or is completed.

strain — (v) to try so hard or do something with so much force that the effort hurts you or makes you, or some part of you, very weak.

succession — following one after another.

technique — a way of doing something that is usually perfected through practice.

More books to read

Aerobics. Working Out (series). Jeff Savage (Silver Burdett)

Courageous Pacers: The Complete Guide to Running, Walking, and Fitness for Kids. Tim Erson (PRO-ACTIV Publications)

Exercise and Your Health. Health Matters (series). Jillian Powell (Raintree Steck-Vaughn)

Feeling Fit. Alicia Martinez (Troll Communications)

Fit for Life. Alexandra Parsons (Watts)

Hatha Yoga for Kids — By Kids. Yogaville Children (Integral Yoga Publications)

Keep Fit. Staying Healthy (series). Miriam Moss (Silver Burdett)

Stay Fit: Build a Strong Body. Catherine Reef (TFC Books)

Staying Healthy: Let's Exercise. Library of Healthy Living (series). A. B. McGinry (Rosen Group)

Weight Lifting. Working Out (series). Jeff Savage (Silver Burdett)

Videos

The American Junior Workout. (Good Times Home Video Corporation)

Fun House Fitness. (Warner Home Video)

Hip Hop Animal Rock Workout Video. (Polygram Records)

Home Exercise for All Ages (Hatha Yoga). (Vision Productions)

Kids-ercise Workout Tape. (I. J. E. Book Publishing/Kid Stuff)

Rope Jumping. (Agency for Instructional Technology)

Web sites

fyiowa.webpoint.com/fitness/index.htm

ificinfo.health.org/brochure/10tipkid.htm

www.fitnesslink.com/changes/kids.htm

www.kidshealth.org/kid/

Due to the dynamic nature of the Internet, some web sites stay current longer than others. To find additional web sites, use a reliable search engine with one or more of the following keywords: *aerobics, breathing, dance, exercise, fitness, health, jogging, yoga.*

Index